Breast Cancer Imaging II

Guest Editors

SANDIP BASU, MBBS (Hons),
DRM, DNB, MNAMS
RAKESH KUMAR, MD
AYŞE MAVİ, MD
ABASS ALAVI, MD,
MD (Hon), PhD (Hon), DSc (Hon)

PET CLINICS

www.pet.theclinics.com

Consulting Editor
ABASS ALAVI, MD,
MD (Hon), PhD (Hon), DSc (Hon)

October 2009 • Volume 4 • Number 4

SAUNDERS an imprint of ELSEVIER, Inc.

W.B. SAUNDERS COMPANY
A Division of Elsevier Inc.

1600 John F. Kennedy Boulevard ● Suite 1800 ● Philadelphia, Pennsylvania 19103-2899

http://www.theclinics.com

PET CLINICS Volume 4, Number 4
October 2009 ISSN 1556-8598, ISBN 10: 1-4377-1402-1, ISBN-13: 978-1-4377-1402-9

Editor: Barton Dudlick

PET Clinics (ISSN 1556-8598) is published quarterly by Elsevier Inc., 360 Park Avenue South, New York, NY 10010-1710. Months of issue are January, April, July, and October. Periodicals postage paid at New York, NY, and additional mailing offices. Subscription prices per year are $196.00 (US individuals), $279.00 (US institutions), $97.00 (US students), $223.00 (Canadian individuals), $312.00 (Canadian institutions), $118.00 (Canadian students), $237.00 (foreign individuals), $312.00 (foreign institutions), and $118.00 (foreign students). To receive student and resident rate, orders must be accompanied by name of affiliated institution, date of term, and the signature of program/residency coordinator on institution letterhead. Orders will be billed at individual rate until proof of status is received. Foreign air speed delivery is included in all Clinics subscription prices. All prices are subject to change without notice. POSTMASTER: Send address changes to PET Clinics, Elsevier Health Sciences Division, Subscription Customer Service, 3251 Riverport Lane, Maryland Heights, MO 63043. **Customer Service: 1-800-654-2452 (U.S. and Canada); 314-447-8871 (outside U.S. and Canada). Fax: 314-447-8029. E-mail: journalscustomerservice-usa@elsevier.com (for print support); journalsonlinesupport-usa@elsevier.com (for online support).**

Reprints. For copies of 100 or more of articles in this publication, please contact the Commercial Reprints Department, Elsevier Inc., 360 Park Avenue South, New York, NY 10010-1710. Tel.: 212-633-3812; Fax: 212-462-1935; E-mail: reprints@elsevier.com.

Printed and bound in the United Kingdom

Transferred to Digital Print 2011

Contributors

CONSULTING EDITOR

ABASS ALAVI, MD, MD (Hon), PhD (Hon), DSc (Hon)
Director of Research Education, Nuclear Medicine Section, Department of Radiology, Hospital of the University of Pennsylvania, Philadelphia, Pennsylvania

GUEST EDITORS

SANDIP BASU, MBBS (Hons), DRM, DNB, MNAMS
Head, Nuclear Medicine Academic Programme, Radiation Medicine Centre (BARC), Tata Memorial Hospital, Parel, Mumbai, India

RAKESH KUMAR, MD
Associate Professor, Department of Nuclear Medicine, All India Institute of Medical Sciences, New Delhi, India

AYŞE MAVİ, MD
Associate Professor, Department of Nuclear Medicine, Yeditepe University Hospital, Istanbul, Turkey

ABASS ALAVI, MD, MD (Hon), PhD (Hon), DSc (Hon)
Director of Research Education, Nuclear Medicine Section, Department of Radiology, Hospital of the University of Pennsylvania, Philadelphia, Pennsylvania

AUTHORS

ABASS ALAVI, MD, MD (Hon), PhD (Hon), DSc (Hon)
Director of Research Education, Nuclear Medicine Section, Department of Radiology, Hospital of the University of Pennsylvania, Philadelphia, Pennsylvania

SANDIP BASU, MBBS (Hons), DRM, DNB, MNAMS
Head, Nuclear Medicine Academic Programme, Radiation Medicine Centre (BARC), Tata Memorial Hospital, Parel, Mumbai, India

FRANÇOIS BÉNARD, MD
Professor, Department of Radiology, University of British Columbia and Centre of Excellence for Functional Cancer Imaging, British Columbia Cancer Agency; BC Cancer Agency Research Centre, British Columbia, Canada

SUSHIL BERIWAL, MD
Associate Professor of Medicine, Department of Radiation Oncology, University of Pittsburgh Cancer Institute, Magee-Womens Hospital of UPMC, Pittsburgh, Pennsylvania

TEVFİK FİKRET ÇERMİK, MD
Associate Professor, Clinic of Nuclear Medicine, Istanbul Education and Research Hospital, Istanbul, Turkey

MADHAVI CHAWLA, MD
Senior Research Associate, Department of Nuclear Medicine, All India Institute of Medical Sciences, New Delhi, India

WILLIAM B. EUBANK, MD
Associate Professor of Radiology, Department
of Radiology, Puget Sound VA Health Care
System, Seattle, Washington

RAKESH KUMAR, MD
Associate Professor, Department of Nuclear
Medicine, All India Institute of Medical
Sciences, New Delhi, India

JEAN H. LEE, MD
Assistant Professor, Department of Radiology,
University of Washington Medical
Center, University of Washington
and Seattle Cancer Care Alliance,
Seattle, Washington

DAVID A. MANKOFF, MD, PhD
Professor of Radiology, Department of
Radiology, University of Washington and
Seattle Cancer Care Alliance, Seattle,
Washington

AYŞE MAVİ, MD
Associate Professor, Department of Nuclear
Medicine, Yeditepe University Hospital,
Istanbul, Turkey

CHRISTOPHER THOMPSON, DSc
Department of Medical Physics, Montreal
Neurological Institute, McGill University,
Montreal, Quebec, Canada

SUSAN WEINSTEIN, MD
Associate Professor, Department of Radiology,
Division of Breast Imaging, University of
Pennsylvania Medical Center, Philadelphia,
Pennsylvania

HABIB ZAIDI, PhD, PD
Division of Nuclear Medicine, Geneva
University Hospital, Geneva,
Switzerland

Contents

Habib Zaidi and Christopher Thompson

Molecular imaging using high-resolution PET instrumentation is now playing a pivotal role in basic and clinical research. The development of optimized detection geometries combined with high-performance detector technologies and compact designs of PET tomographs have become the goal of active research groups in academic and corporate settings. Significant progress has been achieved in the design of commercial PET instrumentation in the last decade allowing a spatial resolution of about 4 to 6 mm to be reached for whole-body imaging, about 2.4 mm for PET cameras dedicated for brain imaging, and submillimeter resolution for female breast, prostate, and small-animal imaging. In particular, significant progress has been made in the design of dedicated positron emission mammography (PEM) units. The initial concept suggested in 1993 consisted of placing 2 planar detectors capable of detecting the 511-keV annihilation photons in a conventional mammography unit. Since that time, many different design paths have been pursued and it will be interesting to see which technologies become the most successful in the future. This paper discusses recent advances in PEM instrumentation and the advantages and challenges of dedicated standalone and dual-modality imaging systems. Future opportunities and the challenges facing the adoption of PEM imaging instrumentation and its role in clinical and research settings are also addressed.

François Bénard and Ayşe Mavi

With advances in gene microarray technologies, the classification of breast cancers has been revised to take into account new information based on common genetic factors that are associated with clinically significant subgroups. At present, breast cancer is divided into 4 major subgroups, Luminal A, Luminal B, HER2/neu positive, and Basal-like. Many breast cancer researchers believe that this classification scheme will change with further subdivision of these categories in various prognostic subgroups. The presence of hormone or growth factor receptors is a key factor in the current classification. Beyond their interest as biomarkers associated with specific subgroups of breast cancer, the expression of receptors in breast cancer has profound therapeutic implications. Given the importance of these receptors in the management of breast cancer, many receptor-binding radiotracers have been developed over the past 30 years. In this article, the current status of receptor-binding radiotracers in breast cancer is reviewed.

Susan Weinstein, Madhavi Chawla, and Rakesh Kumar

Breast cancer is one of the most common cancers in women. Contralateral breast carcinoma is the most common second malignancy in patients with breast carcinoma. Bilateral breast carcinomas exist in 2 forms: synchronous, in which both tumors occur at the same time, or metachronous, in which they occur at different times. When breast cancer is diagnosed, the contralateral breast should be carefully evaluated for a synchronous tumor. Screening for occult contralateral breast cancer is very important on initial cancer diagnosis. The detection and treatment of a synchronous tumor allows for informed surgical decision making, especially if tissue reconstruction is being considered. If chemotherapy is necessary, the patient would only need treatment once for bilateral synchronous cancers, not twice, as with metachronous cancers.

PET/computed tomography–based imaging is a valuable and useful test in the staging and restaging of breast cancer, especially in patients who have recurrent or locally advanced breast cancer. Its greatest clinical applications are in the detection and definition of the extent of recurrent or metastatic disease. However, the potential to improve radiation treatment planning by allowing for the tailoring of comprehensive radiation portals, particularly for locally advanced or recurrent breast cancer, makes it one of the most promising tools in the era of image-guided radiation therapy.

Breast cancer is one of the more responsive solid tumors with a wide range of systemic therapy options. The treatment of newly diagnosed breast cancer is primarily determined by the extent of disease and generally includes surgery, radiation, and chemotherapy. This article discusses the PET and PET-CT modalities for evaluating treatment response in breast cancer.

Whereas ^{18}F-fluorodeoxyglucose (FDG)-PET/computed tomography has proven to be valuable for breast cancer diagnosis and response evaluation, it is likely that PET radiopharmaceuticals beyond FDG will contribute further to the understanding of breast cancer and thereby further direct breast cancer care. Increasingly specific and quantitative approaches will help direct treatment selection from an ever-expanding and increasing array of targeted breast cancer therapies. This article highlights 4 areas of ongoing research where preliminary patient results look promising: (1) tumor perfusion and angiogenesis, (2) drug delivery and transport, (3) tumor receptor imaging, and (4) early response evaluation. For each area, the biologic background is reviewed and early results are highlighted.

This article reviews the promising application of fluorodeoxyglucose–positron emission tomography (FDG-PET) imaging in exploring tumor biology of breast carcinoma based upon the authors' experience and also reviews current literature on this topic. The interest in this novel aspect of breast PET imaging has gained momentum in recent years as more is understood about the molecular subtypes and heterogeneous behavior of breast cancer. With the development of newer targeted therapies, oncologists are realizing the need for a means of accurate prediction and assessment of treatment response early in the course of therapy. Hence the studies on FDG-PET imaging in exploring the tumor biology of breast carcinoma have focused on: tumor histologic subtypes, hormonal receptor expression, disease burden at diagnosis, tumor proliferation index, and other molecular parameters. The correlation of various PET tracer parameters (eg, 15O-water PET-derived blood flow measurements and 18F-FDG–PET derived glucose metabolism rate parameters) is also of considerable interest. To summarize, the utility of FDG-PET/CT imaging on this aspect of breast carcinoma imaging holds considerable promise in disease characterization, and it can be foreseen that it will soon aid in guiding and adapting newer therapeutic regimens.

The precise role of PET/CT (computed tomography) continues to evolve, although 20 years have passed since the first study using ^{18}F 2-Deoxy-2-Fluoro-D-Glucose (FDG)-PET for the assessment of breast cancers. The current whole body PET/CT devices have not achieved adequate accuracy to replace conventional imaging methods and histopathology. Despite the fact that high positive predictive value of FDG-PET and PET/CT in diagnosis of axillary lymph node involvement can avoid sentinel node biopsy in a fraction of metastatic patients, FDG-PET has been shown to be of limited value in staging of axillary lymph node involvement. The current literature demonstrates that FDG-PET and PET/CT are considerably superior compared with conventional methods for the assessment of extra-axillary regional lymph node metastases such as internal mammary and mediastinal lymph nodes. Also, FDG-PET or PET/CT is the preferred method to assess the extent of distant metastatic disease and to diagnose patients with suspicion of recurrent or metastatic disease. Technological developments in positron emission mammography, PET/CT, and PET/MRI have great potential for better diagnosis, staging, and restaging in patients with breast cancer in the near future.

PET Clinics

THE CLINICS ARE NOW AVAILABLE ONLINE!

Access your subscription at:
www.theclinics.com

GOAL STATEMENT

The goal of the *PET Clinics* is to keep practicing radiologists and radiology residents up to date with current clinical practice in positron emission tomography by providing timely articles reviewing the state of the art in patient care.

ACCREDITATION

PET Clinics is planned and implemented in accordance with the Essential Areas and Policies of the Accreditation Council for Continuing Medical Education (ACCME) through the joint sponsorship of the University of Virginia School of Medicine and Elsevier. The University of Virginia School of Medicine is accredited by the ACCME to provide continuing medical education for physicians.

The University of Virginia School of Medicine designates this educational activity for a maximum of 15 *AMA PRA Category 1 Credits*™ for each issue, 60 credits per year. Physicians should only claim credit commensurate with the extent of their participation in the activity.

The American Medical Association has determined that physicians not licensed in the US who participate in this CME activity are eligible for a maximum of 15 *AMA PRA Category 1 Credits*™ for each issue, 60 credits per year.

Category 1 credit can be earned by reading the text material, taking the CME examination online at http://www.theclinics.com/home/cme, and completing the evaluation. After taking the test, you will be required to review any and all incorrect answers. Following completion of the test and evaluation, your credit will be awarded and you may print your certificate.

FACULTY DISCLOSURE/CONFLICT OF INTEREST

The University of Virginia School of Medicine, as an ACCME accredited provider, endorses and strives to comply with the Accreditation Council for Continuing Medical Education (ACCME) Standards of Commercial Support, Commonwealth of Virginia statutes, University of Virginia policies and procedures, and associated federal and private regulations and guidelines on the need for disclosure and monitoring of proprietary and financial interests that may affect the scientific integrity and balance of content delivered in continuing medical education activities under our auspices.

The University of Virginia School of Medicine requires that all CME activities accredited through this institution be developed independently and be scientifically rigorous, balanced and objective in the presentation/discussion of its content, theories and practices.

All authors/editors participating in an accredited CME activity are expected to disclose to the readers relevant financial relationships with commercial entities occurring within the past 12 months (such as grants or research support, employee, consultant, stock holder, member of speakers bureau, etc.). The University of Virginia School of Medicine will employ appropriate mechanisms to resolve potential conflicts of interest to maintain the standards of fair and balanced education to the reader. Questions about specific strategies can be directed to the Office of Continuing Medical Education, University of Virginia School of Medicine, Charlottesville, Virginia.

The faculty and staff of the University of Virginia Office of Continuing Medical Education have no financial affiliations to disclose.

The authors/editors listed below have identified no professional or financial affiliations for themselves or their spouse/partner:

Abass Alavi, MD, MD(Hon), PhD(Hon), DSc(Hon) (Guest Editor); Sandip Basu, MBBS (Hons), DRM, DNB, MNAMS (Guest Editor); François Bénard, MD; Sushil Beriwal, MD; Tevfik Fikret Çermik, MD; Madhavi Chawla, MD; Barton Dudlick (Acquisitions Editor); William B. Eubank, MD; Rakesh Kumar, MD (Guest Editor); Jean H. Lee, MD; Ayşe Mavi, MD (Guest Editor); Patrice Rehm, MD (Test Author); Susan Weinstein, MD; and Habib Zaidi, PhD, PD.

The authors/editors listed below identified the following professional or financial affiliations for themselves or their spouse/partner:

David A. Mankoff, MD, PhD is an industry funded research/investigator for Pfizer and Merck.
Christopher Thompson, DSc is employed by and is a patent holder for Scanwell Systems.

Disclosure of Discussion of Non-FDA Approved Uses for Pharmaceutical Products and/or Medical Devices.
The University of Virginia School of Medicine, as an ACCME provider, requires that all faculty presenters identify and disclose any off-label uses for pharmaceutical and medical device products. The University of Virginia School of Medicine recommends that each physician fully review all the available data on new products or procedures prior to clinical use.

TO ENROLL

To enroll in the PET Clinics Continuing Medical Education program, call customer service at 1-800-654-2452 or visit us online at www.theclinics.com/home/cme. The CME program is available to subscribers for an additional fee of $175.00.

Preface

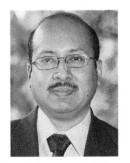

Sandip Basu, MBBS (Hons),
DRM, DNB, MNAMS

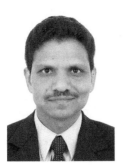

Rakesh Kumar, MD

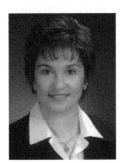

Ayşe Mavi, MD

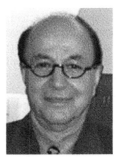

Abass Alavi, MD,
MD (Hon), PhD (Hon),
DSc (Hon)

Guest Editors

THE FUTURE OF FUNCTIONAL IMAGING IN BREAST CARCINOMA

With the rapid changes taking place in modern medicine, foreseeing the future is a perilous exercise. Nevertheless, such predictions allow strategies to be developed that may improve the outcome to some extent. The second part of the *PET Clinics* issue on breast cancer deals with the recent developments in breast cancer imaging, especially with regard to PET/computed tomography (CT), and covers a wide range of topics including technological developments and their potential applications, novel PET tracers beyond fluorodeoxyglucose (FDG), and speculation on the newer applications of FDG-PET imaging beyond diagnostic staging. The outstanding groups of investigators who have contributed to this issue have elegantly portrayed the potential future developments and great versatility of this powerful technology.

With the growing list of treatment regimens and approaches that are available to oncologists, individualizing treatment in patients with cancer has been a hallmark of the modern clinical practice. Therefore, understanding the tumor biology is of utmost importance to select the appropriate therapy in a particular setting. Dr Mankoff and his associates have focused their review on breast cancer imaging on this important topic. The value of understanding this phenomenon in the management of breast cancer has not yet been fully explored. By elucidating the characteristics of tumor perfusion and angiogenesis, tumor receptor status, tumor proliferation index,

multidrug resistance, and novel drug delivery and transport, oncologists may become more successful in selecting the appropriate modes of therapy for furthering patient outcomes as highlighted by this group.

Parallel with the development of novel PET tracers, significant strides have been made toward specialized instruments with the aim of providing high-resolution images of this organ. A spatial resolution of about a few millimeters can now be reached with a specialized positron emission mammography (PEM) unit, which continues to evolve. In their review, Dr Zaidi and his associate highlight the recent advances and the advantages in PEM instrumentation and the challenges in adopting this novel approach in a routine clinical setting.

Assessment of receptor status in breast cancer is of great interest because of its potential prognostic and therapeutic implications. Tumors expressing estrogen and/or progesterone receptors have a higher likelihood of responding to various hormonal therapeutic agents. Currently, the role of several other receptor imaging techniques in characterizing tumor biology is being explored including somatostatin receptor, gastrin-releasing peptide, and neuropeptide Y. The recent observation of a potential link between the estrogen responsiveness of breast cancer and SSTR2 overexpression is of considerable interest to tumor biologists. Dr Bénard and colleague have dealt with this exciting area of breast cancer research in their in-depth review of this topic.

The importance of screening the contralateral breast for occult malignancy in patients with

PET Clin 4 (2009) xi–xii
doi:10.1016/j.cpet.2009.11.002

breast cancer has been emphasized in the recent literature. Detection of tumors in the contralateral side allows for effective surgical decision making, planning for reconstructive surgery, and future systemic therapies. The higher incidence of mortality associated with coincident malignancy in the contralateral breast requires aggressive surgical and medical therapeutic interventions in this population. Hence, selecting and defining the optimal imaging modality to screen both breasts is important at the time of initial diagnosis and at the subsequent follow-up studies. Magnetic resonance imaging and FDG-PET/CT can play an invaluable role in achieving high sensitivity and specificity in this clinical setting. Dr Weinstein and colleagues have placed these 2 powerful tools in perspective in their article. These investigators conclude that a combination of both modalities will provide the necessary screening information to guide subsequent management decisions.

The introduction of PET/CT has provided a major boost to image-guided radiation therapy planning and may become the modality of choice in the near future. Increasingly, radiation oncologists have realized the advantages and the future potential of this powerful approach. Understanding the perspectives of the radiation oncologists and their community is crucial for the success of this promising application. In his review, Dr Beriwal provides the readers with an excellent overview of the rationale and applications of PET/CT imaging for radiation therapy planning in breast carcinoma.

The future applications of FDG-PET imaging extend well beyond disease staging. Early response to therapy has been an area of significant interest in recent years in a wide array of malignancies and breast carcinoma is no exception. Using [^{18}F]FDG-PET allows for predicting response early in the course of therapy and for identifying nonresponders, therefore, serious side effects can be avoided. Such knowledge enables the clinicians to switch to other therapeutic regimens and therapeutic approaches in a timely fashion. Dr Kumar and colleagues have provided a scholarly review of this important application of FDG-PET imaging in breast cancer.

The behavior of breast cancers varies considerably from a slow-growing malignancy that can be managed effectively by locoregional modalities and adjuvant hormone therapy, to rapidly growing incurable disease with widespread metastases at presentation. Functional imaging led by FDG-

PET imaging is playing an increasingly important role in defining tumor biology in this unpredictable malignancy. Dr Basu and colleagues have critically reviewed this new and promising application of FDG-PET imaging based on their own experience at the Hospital of the University of Pennsylvania and have reviewed the current literature on this topic. This article complements that of Çermik and colleagues on the present role of FDG-PET imaging in staging breast carcinoma at diagnosis and at different stages of the disease. FDG-PET imaging seems to have a promising role in assessing the extent of disease throughout the course of this cancer, which would allow optimal planning of various therapeutic interventions.

Finally, we would like to congratulate and express our gratitude to all the authors. They have made painstaking efforts to communicate in a lucid manner what is truly cutting-edge information that will serve as a useful reference source for the next few years. We sincerely hope that our readers will enjoy reading these articles as much as we have.

Sandip Basu, MBBS (Hons), DRM, DNB, MNAMS
Radiation Medicine Centre (BARC)
Tata Memorial Hospital Annex Building
Parel, Mumbai 400012
India

Rakesh Kumar, MD
Department of Nuclear Medicine
All India Institute of Medical Sciences
New Delhi, India

Ayşe Mavi, MD
Department of Nuclear Medicine
Yeditepe University Hospital
Devlet Yolu Ankara Caddesi No: 102/104
Kozyatagi, Istanbul 34752, Turkey

Abass Alavi, MD, MD (Hon), PhD (Hon), DSc (Hon)
Nuclear Medicine Section
Department of Radiology
Hospital of the University of Pennsylvania
3400 Spruce Street
Philadelphia, PA 19104, USA

E-mail addresses:
drsanb@yahoo.com (S. Basu)
rkphulia@hotmail.com (R. Kumar)
aysemavi@yahoo.com (A. Mavi)
abass.alavi@uphs.upenn.edu (A. Alavi)

Evolution and Developments in Instrumentation for Positron Emission Mammography

Habib Zaidi, PhD, PD[a],*, Christopher Thompson, DSc[b]

KEYWORDS

- Positron emission mammography • Molecular imaging
- Instrumentation • Detectors • Breast imaging

THE ROLE OF PET WITHIN THE SPECTRUM OF BREAST IMAGING TECHNIQUES

With the advent of advanced medical imaging technologies, clinical diagnosis is rarely made without imaging. Various structural and functional imaging techniques are used nowadays in the clinic for breast imaging. Conventional diagnostic imaging procedures including x-ray mammography and ultrasound imaging have been the work horse for the last 2 decades. Within the spectrum of macroscopic medical imaging, sensitivity ranges from the detection of millimolar to submillimolar concentrations of contrast medium with structural imaging techniques including computed tomography (CT) and magnetic resonance (MR) imaging, respectively, to picomolar concentrations with molecular imaging techniques including single-photon emission computed tomography (SPECT) and PET, a 10^8 to 10^9 difference.[1]

Radiotracer imaging techniques have gained in popularity during the last decade, particularly with the availability of dedicated breast cameras.[2–4] The use of PET to provide images of glucose metabolism or other physiologic functions of malignant disease is becoming more widespread and whole-body PET (WB-PET) images are now widely used to select the most appropriate therapy in clinical oncology. Since the pioneering work of Dr Wahl on the use of PET for breast cancer imaging,[5] many other reports have been published,[6,7] to cite the first few only. When combined with x-ray CT, PET images provide the equivalent of a "metabolic contrast agent," which serves to highlight the abnormal glucose metabolism in tumors. In a few years, combined PET/CT scanners have become the standard of care in many centers.[8]

PET scanners have a limited spatial resolution compared with structural imaging modalities such as CT and MR. Because the detectability of small tumors leads to earlier diagnosis and treatment, much research and development efforts have focused on improving the spatial resolution of PET. There are both instrumentation and physical factors that degrade the spatial resolution in PET. The fundamental limit is due to the distance positrons travel from the parent nucleus before they lose energy and annihilate with an electron in tissue. Another limitation is caused by the noncollinearity of the pair of annihilation photons, which do not travel away from the point of annihilation at exactly 180 degrees because of the energy of the electron at the time of annihilation. Although this seems to be a fundamental limit in WB-PET, it is much less of a problem in dedicated,

This work was supported by grant no. SNSF 31003A-125246 from the Swiss National Foundation.

[a] Division of Nuclear Medicine, Geneva University Hospital, CH-1211 Geneva, Switzerland
[b] Department of Medical Physics, Montreal Neurological Institute, McGill University, Montreal, QC H3A 2B4, Canada
* Corresponding author.
E-mail address: habib.zaidi@hcuge.ch (H. Zaidi).

PET Clin 4 (2009) 317–327
doi:10.1016/j.cpet.2009.12.002

organ-specific, small, transaxial field-of-view scanners where the detectors are much closer to each other compared with the typical separation needed in WB-PET. The major instrumental limitation is the size of the crystals. Making smaller crystals will improve the spatial resolution at the expense of increased complexity and substantially higher cost. However, if the detectors are placed closer, fewer detectors are required; such instruments dedicated for breast imaging can be produced to provide higher spatial resolution images than those from WB-PET. The factors that contribute to the degradation of the spatial resolution (SR) in PET can be combined as the sum of independent variables in the form:

$$SR = a\sqrt{(d/2)^2 + b^2 + (0.0022D)^2 + r^2}$$

where a is a factor related to the reconstruction algorithm and filter used, d is the crystal width, b combines the effects of light sharing and under-sampling of the image, D is the detector ring diameter, and r is the effective positron range in tissue.

Among the common design factors of PET scanners is the trade-off between spatial resolution, sensitivity, and cost. In the equation above, the crystal width (d) is the variable that balances the cost with the spatial resolution, and the one over which scanner manufacturers have the most control. In WB-PET, moving the detectors closer together is not possible, because this will substantially reduce the patient port and some patients will no longer fit in the scanner. However, this option can be fully exploited in dedicated instruments designed exclusively for small-animal or breast imaging.[9,10]

CLINICAL HISTORY OF POSITRON EMISSION MAMMOGRAPHY

The idea of a dedicated PET scanner for breast imaging was first proposed by Weinberg in 1993, in a United States patent application[11] and a successful Small Business Incentive for Research grant from the US National Institutes of Health (NIH). This was followed by publication of the preliminary results of the first experiments carried out to study the feasibility of the concept.[12] The name positron emission mammography (PEM) was coined to represent this technique. The concept consisted of placing 2 planar detectors capable of detecting the 511-keV annihilation photons in a conventional mammography unit. Placing the breast on a magnification table sometimes used in these instruments provides the possibility of having one detector between the

x-ray tube and the compression plate, and another between the lower aspect of the breast and the x-ray sensor. The 2 detectors move out of the x-ray field for conventional mammography, and move back over and under the breast for the PEM acquisition.[13] This concept predates PET/CT by several years,[14] but the goal was much the same as that of PET/CT as it has evolved today: to provide a coregistered anatomic and functional image in the same procedure with minimal movement of the patient.[8]

An important finding of these first investigations was that a small hyperactive region was just as visible in a superposition of a few near vertical projections as it was in fully reconstructed tomographic images. The experiments were performed in a 15-slice brain scanner on a box phantom containing 4 tubes of various sizes with either no activity or 9.3 times the background. The images were made over different times such that each consecutive image contained half the counts of the previous one. The first paper on PEM provided the basic estimate of the signal-to-noise ratio and the count rate that could be expected from a clinical PEM instrument.[12]

These encouraging results provided the basis for a grant application to the Canadian Breast Cancer Research Initiative. The so-called PEM-1 instrument was built and a preliminary clinical trial was carried out. Because it was concluded that simple back-projection reconstruction provided images with sufficient contrast to identify regions of higher-than-surrounding uptake, the image reconstruction issue was not investigated further as preference was given to providing an almost real-time image display of the PEM image. The goal was to perform the clinical trial using only 75 MBq of [18F]fluorodeoxyglucose (FDG) and an imaging time of 2 minutes per breast (about the time needed to develop an x-ray film in an automatic film processor).

INSTRUMENTATION FOR PEM
Limitations of WB-PET Scanners

An impressive literature exists on the clinical use of large-bore clinical PET scanners in breast imaging for clinical diagnosis, staging and restaging, assessment of response to therapy, and radiation therapy treatment planning.[15–18] A comprehensive overview of the published literature is beyond the scope of this paper.

The detectability of small lesions was affected by the limited spatial resolution of WB-PET systems, reducing the sensitivity and specificity of the technique. Among the various approaches that have been explored to enhance the specificity of FDG-PET for assessing potential malignant lesions is dual-time point imaging, which has been used in assessing various malignancies including those of breast.[19] The theoretic basis for the role of this approach in this setting is that dephosphorylation in tumor cells is either absent or very slow compared with that in normal cells because of their low glucose-6-phosphatase content. This results in a build up of contrast between malignant lesions and the normal tissues with time, which further increases lesion detectability on delayed images. This approach has been tested by several investigators as a potential way to distinguish malignant and benign lesions.[20,21] **Fig. 1** shows the potential of dual-point imaging for improved discrimination between benign and malignant breast cancer. The increase in standardized uptake value (SUV) between the early PET image acquired 1 hour and the delayed image acquired 2 hours post injection is 25%.

The limited spatial resolution of WB-PET systems relative to the size of small lesions also resulted in substantial loss of signal as a result of the partial volume effect. This problem was tackled in many different ways in the context of breast imaging.[22] However, despite the incremental improvement in image quality and resolution, and the enhanced lesion detectability using the various technical approaches developed to address the limitations of imaging small organs such as the breast on WB-PET scanners, emerging clinical

and research applications of molecular breast imaging promise even greater levels of accuracy and precision, and therefore impose more constraints with respect to the intrinsic performance of the PET scanner. Continuous efforts to integrate recent research findings for the design of different geometries and various detector/readout technologies of PET scanners have become the goal of the academic community and nuclear medicine industry. The limited number of studies involving the use of dedicated breast imaging instruments has clearly established the need for PEM to enhance detectability of small tumors.[23] **Fig. 2** compares images of the Derenzo phantom obtained using a general purpose WB-PET system with those obtained using an organ-specific, dedicated, high-resolution PEM scanner. Note the improved spatial resolution on the PEM image, which leads to improved lesion detectability and contrast resolution. **Fig. 3** compares clinical images of a patient with breast cancer obtained using a general-purpose WB-PET system with those obtained using an organ-specific, dedicated, high-resolution PEM scanner showing a mass with increased FDG uptake in the right breast. Similar to the phantom study shown in **Fig. 2**, clinical studies report substantially higher spatial resolution and quantitative accuracy when using the dedicated PEM device. A prospective single-site pilot study designed to evaluate the usefulness of PEM and WB-PET imaging in the surgical management of breast cancer, in which

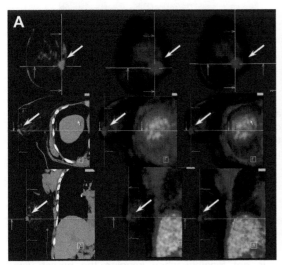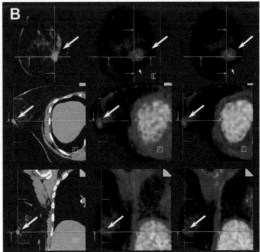

Fig. 1. Illustration of a clinical breast ^{18}F-FDG PET/CT study acquired on a commercial whole-body system showing the potential of dual-point imaging for improved discrimination between benign and malignant breast cancer. The increase in SUV between the early PET image acquired 60 min (*A*) and the delayed image acquired 120 min post-injection (*B*) is 25%. CT, PET, and fused PET/CT images are presented form left to right for axial, sagittal and coronal views.

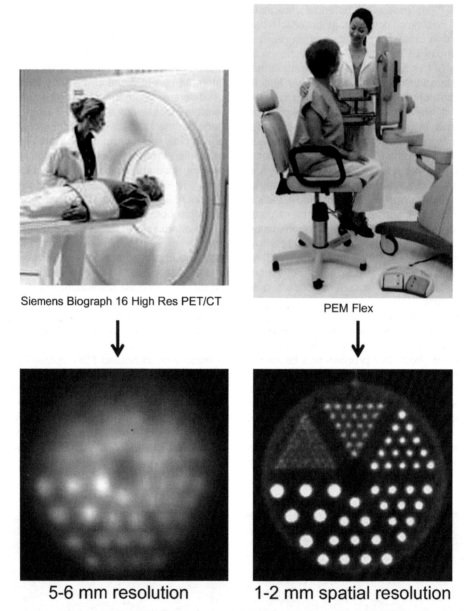

Siemens Biograph 16 High Res PET/CT

PEM Flex

5-6 mm resolution

1-2 mm spatial resolution

Fig. 2. Comparison of phantom images obtained using a general-purpose whole-body PET system with those obtained using an organ-specific, dedicated, high-resolution PEM scanner. Note the improved spatial resolution on the PEM image of the Derenzo phantom, which leads to improved lesion detectability and contrast resolution. (*Courtesy of* Naviscan PET Systems, San Diego, CA, with permission.)

the results from each modality were compared with final surgical histopathology, concluded that PEM had greater sensitivity than WB-PET (92.3% vs 39%).[24]

The Promise of Dedicated PEM Units

In WB-PET scanning, it is a straightforward to over-scan the regions most likely to harbor metastases,

and to overlap the bed positions to compensate for the reduced sensitivity towards the axial ends of each set of slices as a result of the fall-off in three-dimensional sensitivity in the scanner. This is not feasible when imaging the breast using PEM detectors. Even when the detectors are placed very close to the chest wall, some shielding is required. This is a serious problem when imaging small breasts, and for investigations close to the

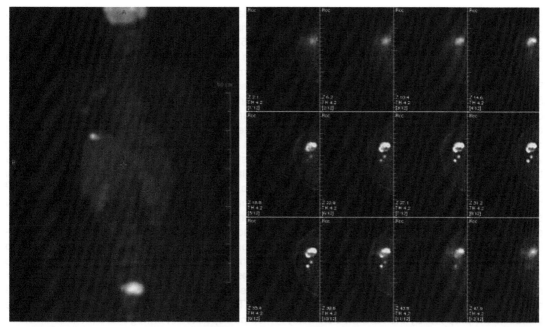

Fig. 3. Comparison of a general purpose whole-body PET scan (*left*) with images obtained using an organ-specific dedicated high resolution PEM scanner (*right*) in a patient with breast cancer. A mass with increased FDG uptake is seen in the right breast. Clinical studies exhibit substantially higher spatial resolution and quantitative accuracy when using the dedicated PEM device. (*Courtesy of* Naviscan PET Systems, San Diego, CA.)

chest wall. Fully three-dimensional PET imaging is always less sensitive towards the axial ends of the field of view because fewer detector pairs can be in coincidence in these regions.

To clearly visualize and accurately quantify the biodistribution of a PET tracer in small structures within the breast requires dedicated high-resolution PET units.[25] In the last 2 decades, much worthwhile research and development efforts have been devoted to the development of dedicated PET scanners for breast imaging. This work has resulted in the development of numerous research prototypes[26–35] and commercially available PEM systems.[36]

Overview of Current PEM Systems

The ultimate performance in spatial resolution, sensitivity, and signal-to-noise ratio of dedicated PEM units can be achieved through careful selection of the design geometry, detector assembly, readout electronics, optimized data acquisition protocols, and image reconstruction algorithms. The rationale in designing dedicated breast versus multipurpose WB-PET scanners is that unlike whole-body imaging where a larger detector ring diameter is needed to accommodate large patients, the size of the female breast is relatively small thus allowing the scanner's diameter to be

reduced and the solid-angle coverage to be increased, leading to higher sensitivity per unit detector volume. A small field-of-view design has the advantage of improving the inherent spatial resolution degradation caused by noncollinearity of the annihilation photons in addition to reducing the overall cost of the PET scanner at the expense of a higher parallax error, hence an image degradation depending on the emission point in the transaxial plane and/or the angle of incidence of the lines of responses. This effect becomes worse when reducing the diameter of the scanner or the size of the crystal's cross-sectional area. This inherent limitation could be coped with by keeping the radial length of the crystal small, typically at values around the attenuation length at 511 keV, which however would strongly compromise the detection efficiency.

Various PEM geometries have been proposed and some of these are currently in use. However, only 1 commercial device has been approved by the Food and Drug Administration (FDA) for clinical use.[37] Almost all have a larger field of view than the first prototype. Complete coverage of the breast while the breast remains in place has become the norm. Various detector arrangements have been proposed, including the classic 2 parallel crystal arrays coupled to position-sensitive photomultipliers (PS-PMTs). One detector is moveable to allow positioning of the breast and for variable compression to suit the patient's anatomy. This geometry was first used in the PEM-1 scanner,[38–40] and later by Smith and colleagues.[41,42] The technique used on the only commercially available PEM Flex Solo scanner (Naviscan PET Systems, San Diego, CA) exploits a pair of linear arrays of detectors that scan across the breast during the examination.[25,36] Another design consists of a boxlike detector array that surrounds the breast, which should allow a more complete reconstruction of the activity within the breast.[43] A similar concept, not yet reduced to practice or implemented in either an experimental or a clinical setting, encloses the breast in a small cylindrical array of detectors with the breast pendant through the hole.[44]

All of these instruments use finely pixelated detectors and a compact geometry designed to reduce the blurring associated with the noncollinearity of the annihilation photons. Of special interest is the proposal by the Lawrence Berkeley National Laboratory group[45] in which the depth at which each annihilation photon is detected in the crystal is also encoded, allowing for a very compact geometry while avoiding the blurring associated with very oblique annihilation photons penetrating the detector. Another PEM prototype consisting of 2 opposing detectors and an array of pixelated (2 × 2 mm^2) YAP (yttrium aluminum perovskit):Ce crystals coupled to position-sensitive photomultiplier tubes was also developed.[31] The Clear-PEM developed by the Crystal Clear

Collaboration at CERN consists of 2 compact and planar detector heads with dimensions 16.5 × 14.5 cm^2 for breast and axilla imaging.[29] This design is based on a fast, segmented, high atomic number detector with depth-of-interaction measurement capabilities.

An alternative design has been developed consisting of a dual-plate PET camera with the 2 plates (10 × 15 cm^2) constructed from arrays of 1 × 1 × 3 mm^3 lutetium oxyorthosilicate (LSO) crystals coupled to silicon position-sensitive avalanche photodiodes (PSAPD).[33] Experimental measurements demonstrated close to 1 mm^3 volumetric spatial resolution, less than 12% energy resolution, and approximately 2 ns coincidence time resolution, whereas Monte Carlo simulations predict a 10% to 15% sensitivity for an 8- to 4-cm panel separation. The same group also investigated the advantages of semiconductor detectors comprising cadmium zinc telluride (CZT) crystal slabs with thin anode and cathode strips deposited in orthogonal directions on either side of each slab, which allows narrower energy window settings.[32] Recently, Raylman and colleagues[34] have developed a high-resolution PEM/tomography imaging and biopsy device (PEM/PET) to detect and guide the biopsy of suspicious breast lesions. The idea is to acquire PET images to detect abnormal focal tracer uptake and limited-angle PEM images that could be used to corroborate the biopsy needle position before tissue sampling. A spatial resolution of 2.01 mm at the center of the field of view was reported.

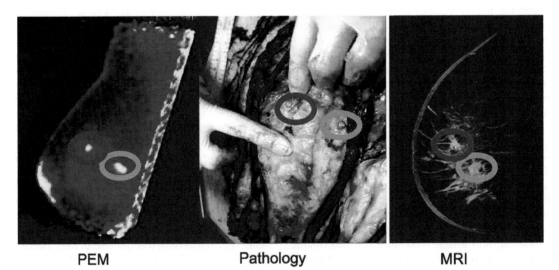

PEM   Pathology   MRI

Fig. 4. A mass with increased FDG uptake in the left breast of a patient with breast cancer. MRI and PEM found 2 IDC lesions not seen by conventional mammography. Ultrasound identified lesion at 10 o'clock. PEM gave a closer estimate of lesion size. More importantly, PEM interpretation time was significantly faster than MRI acquired at 0.6-mm slice thickness which is an important issue for busy diagnostic imaging facilities. (*Courtesy of* Naviscan PET Systems, San Diego, CA.)

The availability of faster scintillation crystals and electronics that made time-of-flight (TOF) PET feasible opened new avenues to partial-ring dedicated PEM scanners without rotation of the detectors.[35] Simulation studies have shown that the contrast recovery coefficient for small hot lesions in a partial-ring scanner is similar to a full-ring non-TOF scanner. In addition, timing resolutions of 600 picoseconds and 300 picoseconds are needed for a two-thirds ring and a half ring scanner, respectively.

CLINICAL RELEVANCE OF PEM

The clinical relevance of this technology and its high diagnostic accuracy for the detection of breast lesions including ductal carcinoma in situ was demonstrated in the recent literature.[25,46,47] A PubMed search (in December 2009) using the term "PEM" resulted in 38 publications ranging from bench studies to large, independent, prospective clinical trials.

The results of the first clinical trial characterizing the clinical performance of PEM was published as early as 1999.[40] During the clinical trial of the PEM-1 scanner, 14 patients were studied including 10 patients who had various breast cancers confirmed by pathologic investigation of the surgically excised specimens. Only 5 of these had a clearly focal uptake (with a mean contrast of 5.8:1 with respect to the surrounding breast tissue). Three other patients were considered PEM-positive based on a significant count-rate asymmetry after accounting for factors such as isotope decay and volume of breast tissue in the field of view and detector separation.[10]

The first report of clinical results from a commercial PEM instrument, the PEM-Flex, were published by Weinberg and colleagues[25] in 2005. They reported on 94 cases performed at 4 different sites during the first year of use of the instrument. Analysis of these cases showed a sensitivity of 93% and a specificity of 83%. Unlike the PEM-1 scanner, the field of view of the commercial device is much larger, 24 × 18 cm versus 5.5 × 6.0 cm. A more sophisticated limited-angle reconstruction algorithm, which produces much clearer three-dimensional images, is also implemented on this system. It also has the ability to scan closer to the chest wall.

A more recent study presented at the 2008 Radiological Society of North America (RSNA) meeting including 208 patients reported that PEM imaging has a similar sensitivity to MR imaging but greater specificity (93% vs 79%).[47] This is consistent with the results reported earlier.[46] In addition, PEM was reported to provide

valuable surgical information for cancer detection and surgical planning.[48] **Fig. 4** demonstrates the good correlation PEM has with both pathology and MRI. In addition, another argument in favour of PEM is the fact that it takes on average only one fourth of the time to interpret the PEM images compared to the time it takes to review the huge number of slices of a breast MRI.

In addition to the improvement in lesion detectability, a substantial improvement of the quantitative accuracy when using PEM compared with WB-PET was reported.[36,49,50] This is an important asset for metabolic characterization of lesions where more accurate estimates of the SUV may assist in discriminating benign and malignant lesions and also improve confidence in assessing response to treatment.

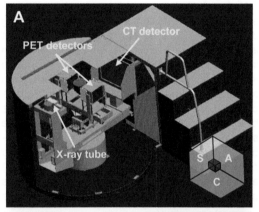

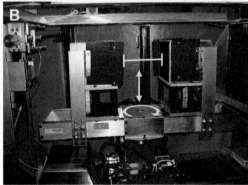

Fig. 5. (A) The dedicated breast PET/CT. The object between the PET detectors shows the approximate position of the patient's breast during scanning. Orientation of positioned patient's coronal (C), sagittal (S), and axial plane (A) are shown in the bottom-right-hand corner. (B) PET gantry allows for control of detector height (*vertical arrow*), separation distance (*horizontal line with end markers*), and rotation (*curved arrow*). (*Reprinted from* Bowen SL, Wu Y, Chaudhari AJ, et al. Initial characterization of a dedicated breast PET/CT scanner during human imaging. J Nucl Med 2009;50:1402; with permission.)

MULTIMODALITY BREAST IMAGING
Software Fusion of Multimodality Breast Imaging

The demand for multimodality imaging arose as a clinical prerequisite given the many positive features it can provide for improving diagnostic and therapeutic procedures. Software-based image registration can be challenging to perform on a routine basis in a clinical setting because it requires compatibility between scanning protocols used by various imaging modalities and outstanding collaboration between various clinical departments. These challenges may be overcome by the use of dual-modality systems described in the following section, however, software-based coregistration offers greater flexibility and might in some cases offer some complementary advantages to hardware-based approaches.[51,52]

Various techniques have been developed to coregister clinical multimodality medical imaging data.[53,54] The coregistration problem in the breast is quite different from the situation in brain imaging. In brain imaging, rigid-body registration involving simple geometric transformations such as translation and rotation to match the 2 image data sets is sufficient in most cases and has been used routinely in clinical settings worldwide since the 1990s. The solution to the image registration problem becomes more complicated particularly when the functional (SPECT or PET) and anatomic (CT or MR imaging) images are acquired in separate sessions on standalone systems, often in different locations and on different days. In this case, geometric relationships between different anatomic regions might be affected by various factors that render the solution difficult to achieve.

Deformable registration (warping) has been introduced as a technique to improve registration accuracy over a larger region of the patient's body. Various deformable image registration techniques have been suggested and used in the context of multimodality breast imaging. However, software-based image registration is still challenging and time consuming in most cases, which limits its use to academic institutions with advanced technical support that can also accommodate the requirements of these procedures (scanning on both modalities on the same day using carefully matched anatomic positioning and respiration protocols).[55,56] Moreover, clinical validation of deformable image registration in the context of breast imaging remains challenging and requires further research and development efforts.[57–60]

Dedicated Breast PET/CT Scanners

The introduction of WB-PET/CT systems in the clinic has revolutionized clinical practice in different ways, particularly in oncology. The use of this technology in the management of patients with breast cancer provides the possibility of correlating metabolic abnormalities observed on PET with patient anatomy, thus improving the

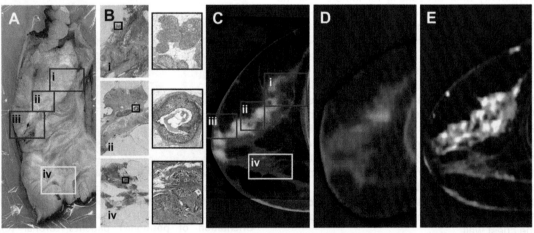

Fig. 6. (A) Sagittal tissue section excised from a mastectomy sample of a clinical study affected breast with 4 areas (*boxes*) of histology performed. (B) Histology tissue slides with magnified regions (*right*, corresponding to black boxes) revealed ductal carcinoma in situ, alone (i, ii) or with intralymphatic invasion (iii, not shown) and benign tissue (iv). Dedicated breast PET/CT (C), WB PET/CT (D), and delayed contrast enhancement MR imaging (E) sagittal image slices corresponding to tissue section (A). Boxes in dedicated breast PET/CT image (C) are at locations approximating those in tissue section (A). PET images (C, D) were windowed between 0% and 60% maximum image intensity. (*Reprinted from* Bowen SL, Wu Y, Chaudhari AJ, et al. Initial characterization of a dedicated breast PET/CT scanner during human imaging. J Nucl Med 2009;50:1406; with permission.)

accuracy of clinical diagnosis with respect to preoperative staging and primary diagnosis, disease restaging, treatment monitoring, and radiation therapy treatment planning.[61,62]

The development of dedicated breast CT units[63,64] paved the way for the introduction of high-resolution PET/CT systems dedicated for the breast with the aim of achieving improved spatial resolution and sensitivity compared with WB-PET systems. One such prototype consisting of an LSO-based dual-planar head PET camera (crystal size, $3 \times 3 \times 20$ mm^3) and 768-slice cone-beam CT was designed, fabricated, and tested at the University of California, Davis, CA, USA (Fig. 5).[65] The average spatial resolution obtained using a line source in warm background using maximum a posteriori (MAP) reconstruction was 2.5 mm; a peak sensitivity of 1.6% was measured at the center of the field of view. Preliminary results from a clinical trial demonstrate the potential of this technology, which clearly visualized the three-dimensional extent of suspected lesions in patients with cancer confirmed by biopsy.[66] Fig. 6 shows a clinical study highlighting the improvement in image quality and contrast resolution when using dedicated breast PET/CT compared with WB-PET/CT.

Other combinations of imaging modalities for breast imaging have also been explored in academic settings including ultrasound (US)-MR,[67] US-mammography,[68] and PET-MR.[69,70] It is not clear if these technologies will find their way to the clinic in the near future and gain popularity as PET/CT did, but the future of multimodality breast imaging is certainly bright and novel emerging hybrid imaging technologies will certainly influence clinical care.

SUMMARY AND FUTURE PERSPECTIVES

Although WB-PET has the potential to detect distant spread of breast cancer, dedicated PEM systems offer a higher spatial resolution and sensitivity, and as such enhance the detectability of small-sized lesions. Following approval of PEM technology by the FDA, many facilities acquired this technology and are now gathering clinical experience through clinical trials.

The major limitation of early PEM instruments was their small field of view and reduced sensitivity near the chest wall. The field of view was limited by the PS-PMTs available in the early 1990s. Recent demands for these devices and their deployment in small-animal PET scanners, has led to much improvement in uniformity and the ability to image much closer to the edge without serious distortion. Now instruments like the PEM Flex Solo are able to

capitalize on the advances in photon sensors. The problem of sensitivity loss near the edges of the field of view is intrinsic to three-dimensional PET acquisitions. During the early stages of PEM development this was not considered seriously enough. Now that it has been widely recognized, the situation has been improved using higher density, thinner shielding, better PMTs, and improved geometry. The effective field of view is at least 3 cm closer to the chest in the latest instruments than in the first prototype.

It is expected that PEM will play a pivotal role for screening high-risk patients and in preoperative surgical staging of patients with recent cancer diagnosis. This technology is not intended to replace conventional mammography as a screening tool, but will likely operate as a complementary molecular imaging tool similar to breast MR imaging.

REFERENCES

1. Jones T. Molecular imaging with PET – the future challenges. Br J Radiol 2002;75:6S–15.
2. Brzymialkiewicz CN, Tornai MP, McKinley RL, et al. Performance of dedicated emission mammotomography for various breast shapes and sizes. Phys Med Biol 2006;51:5051–64.
3. Spanu A, Chessa F, Sanna D, et al. Scintimammography with a high resolution dedicated breast camera in comparison with SPECT/CT in primary breast cancer detection. Q J Nucl Med Mol Imaging 2009;53:271–80.
4. Lee JH, Rosen EL, Mankoff DA. The role of radiotracer imaging in the diagnosis and management of patients with breast cancer: part 2–response to therapy, other indications, and future directions. J Nucl Med 2009;50:738–48.
5. Wahl RL, Cody RL, Hutchins GD, et al. Primary and metastatic breast carcinoma: initial clinical evaluation with PET with the radiolabeled glucose analogue 2-F-18-fluoro-2-deoxy-D-glucose. Radiology 1991;179:765–70.
6. Adler LP, Crowe JP, al-Kaisi NK, et al. Evaluation of breast masses and axillary lymph nodes with F-18 2-deoxy-2-fluoro-D-glucose PET. Radiology 1993;187:743–50.
7. Avril N, Schelling M, Dose J, et al. Utility of PET in breast cancer. Clin Positron Imaging 1999;2:261–71.
8. Townsend DW. Dual-modality imaging: combining anatomy and function. J Nucl Med 2008;49:938–55.
9. Moses WW, Qi J. Instrumentation optimization for positron emission mammography. Nucl Instrum Methods A 2004;527:76–82.
10. Thompson C. Instrumentation for positron emission mammography. PET Clin 2006;1:33–8.
11. Weinberg IN. Dedicated apparatus and method for emission mammography. US Patent 5252830, 1993.

12. Thompson CJ, Murthy K, Weinberg IN, et al. Feasibility study for positron emission mammography. Med Phys 1994;21:529–38.

13. Thompson CJ, Murthy K, Picard Y, et al. Positron emission mammography (PEM): a promising technique for detecting breast cancer. IEEE Trans Nucl Sci 1995;42:1012–7.

14. Bergman AM, Thompson CJ, Murthy K, et al. Technique to obtain positron emission mammography images in registration with x-ray mammograms. Med Phys 1998;25:2119–29.

15. Groheux D, Hindié E, Rubello D, et al. Should FDG PET/CT be used for the initial staging of breast cancer? Eur J Nucl Med Mol Imaging 2009;36:1539–42.

16. Heusner T, Kuemmel S, Hahn S, et al. Diagnostic value of full-dose FDG PET/CT for axillary lymph node staging in breast cancer patients. Eur J Nucl Med Mol Imaging 2009;36:1543–50.

17. Duch J, Fuster D, Muñoz M, et al. ^{18}F-FDG PET/CT for early prediction of response to neoadjuvant chemotherapy in breast cancer. Eur J Nucl Med Mol Imaging 2009;36:1551–7.

18. Avril N, Sassen S, Roylance R. Response to therapy in breast cancer. J Nucl Med 2009;1(50 Suppl 1): 55S–63S.

19. Basu S, Zaidi H, Alavi A. Clinical and research applications of quantitative PET imaging. PET Clinics 2007;2:161–72.

20. Kumar R, Loving VA, Chauhan A, et al. Potential of dual-time-point imaging to improve breast cancer diagnosis with ^{18}F-FDG PET. J Nucl Med 2005;46: 1819–24.

21. Mavi A, Urhan M, Yu JQ, et al. Dual time point ^{18}F-FDG PET imaging detects breast cancer with high sensitivity and correlates well with histologic subtypes. J Nucl Med 2006;47:1440–6.

22. Avril N, Bense S, Ziegler SI, et al. Breast imaging with fluorine-18-FDG PET: quantitative image analysis. J Nucl Med 1997;38:1186–91.

23. Weinberg IN. Applications for positron emission mammography. Phys Med 2006;21(Suppl 1):132–7.

24. Schilling K. High-resolution positron emission mammography in breast cancer [abstract]. J Nucl Med 2007;48:139.

25. Weinberg IN, Beylin D, Zavarzin V, et al. Positron emission mammography: high-resolution biochemical breast imaging. Technol Cancer Res Treat 2005;4:55–60.

26. Freifelder R, Karp JS. Dedicated PET scanners for breast imaging. Phys Med Biol 1997;42:2463–80.

27. Doshi NK, Silverman RW, Shao Y, et al. maxPET, a dedicated mammary and axillary region PET imaging system for breast cancer. IEEE Trans Nucl Sci 2001;48:811–5.

28. Wang G-C, Huber JS, Moses WW, et al. Characterization of the LBNL PEM camera. IEEE Trans Nucl Sci 2006;53:1129–35.

29. Abreu MC, Aguiar D, Albuquerque E, et al. Clear-PEM: a PET imaging system dedicated to breast cancer diagnostics. Nucl Instr Meth A 2007;571:81–4.

30. Raylman RR, Majewski S, Wojcik R, et al. The potential role of positron emission mammography for detection of breast cancer. A phantom study. Med Phys 2000;27:1943–54.

31. Belcari N, Camarda M, Del Guerra A, et al. Detector development for a novel positron emission mammography scanner based on YAP:Ce crystals. Nucl Instr Meth A 2004;525:258–62.

32. Levin CS, Foudray AM, Habte F. Impact of high energy resolution detectors on the performance of a PET system dedicated to breast cancer imaging. Phys Med 2006;21(Suppl 1):28–34.

33. Zhang J, Olcott PD, Chinn G, et al. Study of the performance of a novel 1 mm resolution dual-panel PET camera design dedicated to breast cancer imaging using Monte Carlo simulation. Med Phys 2007;34:689–702.

34. Raylman RR, Majewski S, Smith MF, et al. The positron emission mammography/tomography breast imaging and biopsy system (PEM/PET): design, construction and phantom-based measurements. Phys Med Biol 2008;53:637–53.

35. Surti S, Karp JS. Design considerations for a limited angle, dedicated breast, TOF PET scanner. Phys Med Biol 2008;53:2911–21.

36. MacDonald L, Edwards J, Lewellen T, et al. Clinical imaging characteristics of the positron emission mammography camera: PEM Flex Solo II. J Nucl Med 2009;50:1666–75.

37. Samson D, Redding Flamm C, Aronson N. FDG positron emission tomography for evaluating breast cancer. Chicago: Blue Cross and Blue Shield Association; 2001. Available at: http://www.cms.hhs.gov/coverage/download/id71.pdf.

38. Robar JL, Thompson CJ, Murthy K, et al. Construction and calibration of detectors for high-resolution metabolic breast cancer imaging. Nucl Instr Meth A 1997;392:402–6.

39. Murthy K, Aznar M, Bergman AM, et al. Positron emission mammographic instrument: initial results. Radiology 2000;215:280–5.

40. Murthy K, Aznar M, Thompson CJ, et al. Results of preliminary clinical trials of the positron emission mammography system PEM-I: a dedicated breast imaging system producing glucose metabolic images using FDG. J Nucl Med 2000;41:1851–8.

41. Smith MF, Majewski S, Weisenberger AG, et al. Analysis of factors affecting positron emission mammography (PEM) image formation. IEEE Trans Nucl Sci 2003;50:53–9.

42. Smith MF, Raylman RR, Majewski S, et al. Positron emission mammography with tomographic acquisition using dual planar detectors: initial evaluations. Phys Med Biol 2004;49:2437–52.

43. Huber JS, Choong WS, Wang J, et al. Development of the LBNL positron emission mammography camera. IEEE Trans Nucl Sci 2003;50:1650–3.

44. Karimian A, Thompson CJ, Sarkar S, et al. CYBPET: a cylindrical PET system for breast imaging. Nucl Instr Meth A 2005;545:427–35.

45. Huber JS, Moses WW, Wang GC, et al. A retrospective on the LBNL PEM project. Phys Med 2006; 21(Suppl 1):60–3.

46. Berg WA, Weinberg IN, Narayanan D, et al. High-resolution fluorodeoxyglucose positron emission tomography with compression ("positron emission mammography") is highly accurate in depicting primary breast cancer. Breast J 2006;12:309–23.

47. Schilling K, Narayanan D, Kalinyak J. Breast series: identification and management of the patient at high risk for breast cancer. Effect of breast density, menopausal status, and hormone use in high resolution positron emission mammography abstract. RSNA meeting. Chicago, November 30 to December 5, 2008.

48. Tafra L, Cheng Z, Uddo J, et al. Pilot clinical trial of ^{18}F-fluorodeoxyglucose positron-emission mammography in the surgical management of breast cancer. Am J Surg 2005;190:628–32.

49. Wollenweber SD, Williams RC, Beylin D, et al. Investigation of the quantitative capabilities of a positron emission mammography system. IEEE Nuclear Science Symposium Conference Record 2004;4: 2393–5.

50. Raylman RR, Smith MF, Kinahan PE, et al. Quantification of radiotracer uptake with a dedicated breast PET imaging system. Med Phys 2008;35:4989–97.

51. Pietrzyk U. Does PET/CT render software fusion obsolete? Nuklearmedizin 2005;44:S13–7.

52. Weigert M, Pietrzyk U, Muller S, et al. Whole-body PET/CT imaging: combining software- and hardware-based co-registration. Z Med Phys 2008;18:59–66.

53. Maintz JB, Viergever MA. A survey of medical image registration. Med Image Anal 1998;2:1–36.

54. Pluim JP, Maintz JB, Viergever MA. Mutual-information-based registration of medical images: a survey. IEEE Trans Med Imaging 2003;22:986–1004.

55. Krishnasetty V, Fischman AJ, Halpern EL, et al. Comparison of alignment of computer-registered data sets: combined PET/CT versus independent PET and CT of the thorax. Radiology 2005;237:635–9.

56. Slomka PJ. Software approach to merging molecular with anatomic information. J Nucl Med 2004; 45(Suppl 1):36S–45S.

57. Schnabel JA, Tanner C, Castellano-Smith AD, et al. Validation of nonrigid image registration using finite-element methods: application to breast MR images. IEEE Trans Med Imaging 2003;22: 238–47.

58. Crum WR, Tanner C, Hawkes DJ. Anisotropic multi-scale fluid registration: evaluation in magnetic resonance breast imaging. Phys Med Biol 2005;50(21): 5153–74.

59. Rohlfing T, Maurer CR, Bluemke DA, et al. Volume-preserving nonrigid registration of MR breast images using free-form deformation with an incompressibility constraint. IEEE Trans Med Imaging 2003;22:730–41.

60. Krol A, Unlu MZ, Baum KG, et al. MRI/PET nonrigid breast-image registration using skin fiducial markers. Phys Med 2006;21(Suppl 1):39–43.

61. Zangheri B, Messa C, Picchio M, et al. PET/CT and breast cancer. Eur J Nucl Med Mol Imaging 2004; 31:S135–42.

62. Rosen EL, Eubank WB, Mankoff DA. FDG PET, PET/CT, and breast cancer imaging. Radiographics 2007;27(Suppl 1):S215–29.

63. Boone JM, Lindfors KK. Breast CT: potential for breast cancer screening and diagnosis. Future Oncol 2006;2:351–6.

64. Lindfors KK, Boone JM, Nelson TR, et al. Dedicated breast CT: initial clinical experience. Radiology 2008;246:725–33.

65. Wu Y, Bowen SL, Yang K, et al. PET characteristics of a dedicated breast PET/CT scanner prototype. Phys Med Biol 2009;54:4273–87.

66. Bowen SL, Wu Y, Chaudhari AJ, et al. Initial characterization of a dedicated breast PET/CT scanner during human imaging. J Nucl Med 2009;50:1401–8.

67. Tang AM, Kacher DF, Lam EY, et al. Simultaneous ultrasound and MRI system for breast biopsy: compatibility assessment and demonstration in a dual modality phantom. IEEE Trans Med Imaging 2008;27:247–54.

68. Sinha SP, Goodsitt MM, Roubidoux MA, et al. Automated ultrasound scanning on a dual-modality breast imaging system: coverage and motion issues and solutions. J Ultrasound Med 2007;26: 645–55.

69. Ravindranath B, Maramraju SH, Junnarkar SS, et al. A simultaneous PET/MRI breast scanner based on the RatCAP. IEEE Nuclear Science Symposium Conference Record 2008;4650–5.

70. Ravindranath B, Junnarkar SS, Purschke ML, et al. Results from prototype II of the BNL simultaneous PET-MRI dedicated breast scanner. IEEE Nuclear Science Symposium Conference Record, in press.

Receptor Imaging in Patients with Breast Cancer

François Bénard, MD[a],*, Ayşe Mavi, MD[b]

KEYWORDS
• Breast cancer • Receptor imaging
• Growth factor receptors • Hormone receptors

Breast cancer is a malignancy that is increasingly viewed as a heterogeneous group of diseases with varying biologic behaviors. The behavior of breast cancers can range from a slowly progressive malignancy, readily managed by local treatment and adjuvant hormone therapy, to rapidly growing, incurable, and aggressive breast cancers with widespread metastases at presentation. With advances in gene microarray technologies, the classification of breast cancers has been revised to take into account new information based on common genetic factors that are associated with clinically significant subgroups. At present, breast cancer is divided into 4 major subgroups: Luminal A, Luminal B, HER2/neu positive, and Basal-like.[1,2] Many breast cancer researchers believe that this classification scheme will change with further subdivision of these categories in various prognostic subgroups. The presence of hormone or growth factor receptors is a key factor in the current classification. Luminal A and B cancers express hormone receptors, the HER2/neu group is defined by the expression of this oncogene, irrespective of the steroid hormone receptor status, and the basal subgroup is defined by the complete absence of estrogen receptors (ER), progesterone receptors (PR), or the HER2/neu oncogene, along with specific cell markers associated with the basal subtype.[1]

Beyond their interest as biomarkers associated with specific subgroups of breast cancer, the expression of receptors in breast cancer has profound therapeutic implications. Women expressing ER or PR have a much higher likelihood of responding to various hormone therapy agents, which include partial antagonists (tamoxifen), progesterone derivatives (megestrol acetate), steroidal aromatase inhibitors (exemestane), nonsteroidal aromatase inhibitors (anastrozole, letrozole), and pure estrogen antagonists (fulvestrant).[3] Aromatase inhibitors are typically preferred in the adjuvant setting nowadays.[4] Women who develop resistance to one class of hormone therapy drugs may respond to a drug from a different class. Breast cancers that express the HER2/neu oncogene respond to immunotherapy with trastuzumab (Herceptin). Whereas HER2/neu overexpression used to be associated with rapid progression and an unfavorable prognosis,[5] the use of trastuzumab in the adjuvant setting profoundly improves the prognosis of this group of breast cancer patients.[6] Basal breast cancers may be sensitive to hormone therapy, but once this group of breast cancers reaches metastatic status the prognosis is usually poor, with progressive resistance to various chemotherapy drugs.[7]

Given the importance of these receptors in the management of breast cancer, many receptor-binding radiotracers have been developed over the past 30 years. So far, none have reached widespread clinical acceptance, in part due to

[a] Department of Radiology, University of British Columbia and Centre of Excellence for Functional Cancer Imaging, BC Cancer Agency Research Centre, British Columbia Cancer Agency, 675 West 10th Avenue West, Vancouver, BC V5Z 1L3, Canada
[b] Department of Nuclear Medicine, Yeditepe University Hospital, Devlet Yolu Ankara Street No: 102/104 Kozyatagi 34752, Istanbul, Turkey
* Corresponding author.
E-mail address: fbenard@bccrc.ca (F. Bénard).

PET Clin 4 (2009) 329–341
doi:10.1016/j.cpet.2009.10.004

challenges in clinical translation and conducting multicenter trials with these radiotracers. In this article, the current status of receptor-binding radiotracers in breast cancer is reviewed.

STEROID HORMONE RECEPTOR IMAGING

The presence of ERs and PRs is predictive of a successful response to hormone therapy. Whereas ER expression alone is associated with a favorable response to hormone therapy, PR expression has been shown to have additional value to predict a successful response to tamoxifen.[8] The presence of both receptors is more predictive than either receptor alone. The initial techniques for measuring ER and PR expression relied on radiotracer-based in vitro ligand-binding assays[9] or enzyme immunoassays,[10] which required substantial amounts of tissue for receptor characterization. These techniques were replaced several years ago by immunohistochemistry, which can be performed on core-needle biopsy samples. The reliability of immunohistochemistry ER and PR assays has been shown as comparable with competitive binding assays,[11,12] but quality control is important. Lack of standardization and proper quality control can result in significant discrepancies in ER/PR characterization across laboratories.[13,14] In addition, these methods are subject to sampling error. In general, however, immunohistochemistry is considered reliable for the determination of ER/PR status at diagnosis, and imaging plays little role in this setting.

The receptor expression can change at the time of systematic relapse and during treatment,[15,16] and metastases may differ from the primary tumor in ER/PR levels.[17] Thus, additional biopsies are needed to know the actual receptor status at the time of relapse to achieve second- or third-line treatment. In patients with acquired resistance to endocrine treatment, determining the actual ER status by biopsies is often difficult to perform, because systemic metastases can be difficult to access due to their location and receptor status can be discordant in 20% to 30% of simultaneous biopsies from a single patient.[17,18] Conversion rates from ER-positive to ER-negative status of 29% to 31% have been reported, while conversion rates from ER-negative to ER-positive status have also been reported in a significant proportion (12%–33%) of cases between the assessment of ER expression in the primary tumor and relapse.[18,19] Heterogeneity between the primary site and metastases is also a well documented phenomenon.[20] Steroid receptor imaging can measure receptor expression across various metastatic sites and assess receptor expression

in recurrent breast cancers,[21–23] which is likely to be beneficial when tissue diagnosis is difficult or requires invasive procedures.

Estrogen Receptors

A review of estrogen receptor biology and various ER binding ligands can be found in an article by Beauregard and colleagues.[24] Hochberg[25] developed the first ER imaging radiotracer for nuclear medicine, [^{125}I]estradiol. In a study conducted on 29 women with breast cancer, the value of 16α-[^{123}I]iodo-17β-estradiol imaging in determining the ER status was evaluated.[26] Imaging of tumors in the abdomen was particularly difficult due to the rapid clearance of tracer from blood via the liver, gallbladder, and intestines. ER-positive tumors in the thorax could be correctly identified in 7 out of 9 patients. The density of the ER in the tumor was relatively low in the 2 false-negative cases. In all 12 patients with ER-negative lesions, no tumors were detected. In a follow up study, an overall sensitivity of 66% (20/30) and an overall specificity of 92% (11/12) detection of ER-positive tumors were reported.[27] Several other iodinated estrogen receptor derivatives were then developed, including methoxy-iodo-vinyl-estradiol ([^{123}I]Z-MIVE), which was successfully used to image ER in clinical studies.[28–36]

[^{18}F]Fluoroestradiol ([^{18}F]FES) was developed jointly by the research groups of Welch and Katzenellenbogen at the Mallinckrodt Institute of Radiology in St. Louis.[37] This radiotracer showed high affinity for the estrogen receptor and good uterus uptake in preclinical models. Although rapidly metabolized and conjugated, [^{18}F]FES uptake correlates well with breast cancer ER content when using either competitive binding assays or immunohistochemistry.[21,38] [^{18}F]FES binding to sex-hormone binding globulin (SHBG)[39] partially protects it from metabolism by hepatocytes.[40] [^{18}F]FES can be safely used in humans, with an acceptable radiation dosimetry.[41]

In addition to receptor density, [^{18}F]FES PET can also measure receptor occupancy. In vivo optimization of the drug dosing schedule can be achieved by competition experiments using tamoxifen.[42] [^{18}F]FES is a subtype selective tracer. Studies in ERα and in ERβ show that [^{18}F]FES preferentially binds to the α-subtype of the ER receptor.[43]

Detecting low levels of ER expression in breast cancer with [^{18}F]FES may be challenging, as such low levels may still be clinically relevant in predicting a favorable response to hormone therapy.[38] Other derivatives of [^{18}F]FES have been developed. 16β-Fluoromoxestrol showed promising results in preclinical studies but did not seem to work in a human study in women with breast cancer.[40,44] 4-Fluoro-11β-methoxy-fluoroestradiol ([18F]4F-MFES), an [18F]FES analogue designed for lower nonspecific binding and improved metabolic stability, showed promise in preclinical studies, with very high uterus and tumor to background ratios, despite a slightly lower binding affinity to ER than [18F]FES.[45,46] A phase I study conducted in healthy patients for dosimetry showed good uterus uptake of [18F]4F-MFES despite a documented lack of SHBG binding, with very fast blood clearance and acceptable radiation dosimetry.[47] Whether [18F]4F-MFES provides higher tumor to background ratios compared with [18F]FES remains to be determined by a comparative clinical study. At present, [18F]FES remains the radiopharmaceutical of choice for ER imaging in clinical trials. The radiochemical synthesis is relatively easy to perform, with batches of high specific activity.[48] Immediate precursors for radiolabeling are available commercially, and a few clinical studies have shown the efficacy of this agent to predict response to hormone therapy.

Mintun and colleagues[49] first showed the good correlation between in vitro receptor ER assays and uptake of [18F]FES. The same group showed good sensitivity of ER imaging in detecting uptake in primary tumors and metastases in a subsequent study.[23] In a study of 43 patients, a sensitivity of 76% and specificity of 100% of [18F]FES PET was found when results were compared with immunohistochemical assays for ER expression.[50] Mortimer and colleagues[51] also showed that high [18F]FES uptake (defined as a standardized uptake value [SUV] >2.0) was predictive of response to tamoxifen in 40 women with recurrent breast carcinoma. These investigators observed, however, a considerable overlap between responders and nonresponders in that series, in particular with patients with borderline uptake of [18F]FES. A successful response to tamoxifen was associated with reduction of [18F]FES uptake and a flare reaction characterized by increased [18F]Fluorodeoxyglucose ([18F]FDG) uptake after 7 to 10 days of tamoxifen treatment. Given the impressive results observed with the metabolic flare, the same group repeated a study in 51 women with recurrent breast cancer, most of whom had received prior endocrine treatment.[52] Baseline [18F]FES and [18F]FDG PET scans were obtained. An [18F]FDG PET scan was repeated 24 hours after administration of 30 mg of estradiol challenge. Both a metabolic response (12% increase or more in tumor [18F]FDG uptake) and the baseline [18F]FES uptake were predictive of successful response to hormone therapy, defined as stable disease or partial and complete responses. In this study the [18F]FES cutoff had been determined by a prior study, and the percent increase of [18F]FDG uptake was optimized by receiver operating characteristic analysis performed on the same data set as for the response analysis. Many patients with positive [18F]FES scans (defined again as [18F]FES SUV >2.0) did not respond to hormone therapy. Although the [18F]FDG metabolic flare was predictive of survival, these investigators did not note improved survival in women with high [18F]FES uptake.

Linden and colleagues[53] evaluated 47 patients treated with hormone therapy. This study was a retrospective analysis of patients accrued in 3 clinical trials at the University of Washington. The patients underwent a baseline [18F]FES PET scan before or shortly after hormone therapy initiation, and clinical response was assessed after 6 months. In this study, an objective response was defined as either a partial (PR) or complete response (CR). Patients with stable disease (SD) (usually considered part of the group of patients with a clinical benefit in breast cancer) were considered nonresponders. Most patients were treated with aromatase inhibitors (36/47 cases; 77%). Six patients (13%) were treated with fulvestrant and an aromatase inhibitor. Five patients were treated with tamoxifen alone. Some patients with HER-2/neu overexpression were also treated with trastuzumab. None of the patients with low [18F]FES uptake (SUV cutoff 1.5) responded to hormone therapy, while 34% with a SUV higher than 1.5 responded.

[18F]FES has an initial widespread distribution and crosses the blood-brain barrier. [18F]FES is rapidly metabolized by the liver and is eliminated by both urinary and biliary excretion, with intense accumulation in gallbladder and gut. Liver uptake is high, hindering detection of liver metastases, which may appear as hypoactive ("cold") spots. There is low background activity in the lungs, breast, bones, and other soft tissue. Uptake in the veins draining the injection site is commonly observed. Foci of inflammation can have mild nonspecific [18F]FES uptake. ER-positive tumors usually are seen clearly, but low tumor to background ratios can be observed in cancers with borderline ER positivity.[53] An [18F]FDG PET scan is usually required to establish a map of active metastases for comparison with the [18F]FES images. This scan also helps in the identification of receptor expression heterogeneity, with some [18F]FES negative lesions being identified by [18F]FDG uptake (Fig. 1). In contrast, [18F]FES uptake can also be identified in breast cancer metastases that remain unseen on [18F]FDG scans.

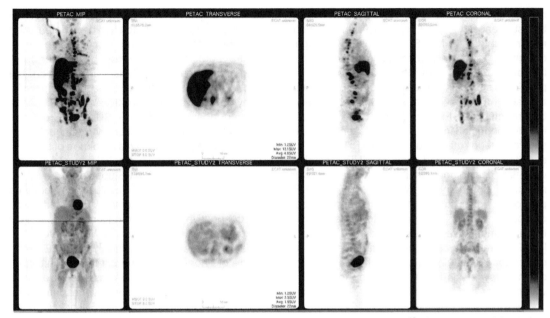

Fig. 1. Patient with metastatic breast cancer on aromatase inhibitor therapy. The ^{18}F-fluoroestradiol (FES) scan (*upper panel*) shows multiple bone metastases with high expression of estrogen receptors. Intense liver uptake is a normal finding due to hepatobiliary excretion of ^{18}F-FES. The lower panel shows the contemporary ^{18}F-FDG scan, with relatively low tracer uptake in the bone metastases due to the effects of endocrine therapy.

[18F]FES was discovered more than 25 years ago, but this tracer has never made any major inroads into routine clinical practice. This failure is partly due to the limited number of clinical trials on the clinical use of [18F]FES, conducted in small groups of patients. Hormone therapy drugs have been validated in large multicenter trials. Given the acceptable toxicity of aromatase inhibitors, tamoxifen, and fulvestrant, most oncologists feel comfortable trying these drugs for a few weeks to months in patients who present with a relapse if the primary tumor was ER-positive. Furthermore, some patients with positive [18F]FES scans may still resist hormone therapy through mechanisms other than loss of ER expression.

The use of an estradiol challenge requires 2 [18F]FDG scans,[52] which is equivalent to the [18F]FDG and [18F]FES scan combination. Administering high doses of estradiol in ER-positive breast cancers may not be acceptable to some patients or physicians, but this compelling approach warrants further evaluation in clinical trials. The cost-effectiveness of these approaches has not been explored in a comparison with the cost of ineffective hormone therapy drugs and delayed treatment. Although [18F]FES imaging can be a useful troubleshooting tool in particular clinical instances, the current data remain limited to justify using this tool in routine clinical practice. Hormone therapy (aromatase inhibitors and fulvestrant, in particular) is not inexpensive, and the consequences of delayed appropriate treatment (typically 6 months are required to assess response) are hard to quantify. Larger trials with a population of women with recurrent breast cancer would be useful to assess whether estrogen receptor imaging can contribute to improve clinical management.

Progesterone Receptors

The PR is the target for treatment with progesterone-derived drugs. Imaging of the PR could influence treatment evaluation in breast cancer. The expression of the PR is estrogen dependent. Progesterone receptors are expressed in response to DNA estrogen response elements, and have additional predictive value on a successful response to hormone therapy to ER positivity.[8] Therefore, PR imaging may also be useful in monitoring the estrogen responsiveness during ER-mediated treatment.

Unfortunately, there are currently no suitable tracers for imaging of PR expression in humans. Only a few tracers for PR imaging have been investigated, with disappointing results. For PET, early studies with the tracer 21-[18F]fluoro-16α-ethyl-19-norprogesterone ([18F]FENP) showed promising results in animal studies.[54] However, the results could not be replicated in humans due to low target to background ratios and metabolic problems.[55,56] [18F]FENP was tested in 8 patients with primary breast carcinoma, and detected only half of PR-positive tumors. To overcome this problem several other progesterone derivatives have been proposed, labeled with [123/125]I, ^{99m}Tc, [77]Br, and [18]F. These compounds have not yet been tested on humans.[57,58]

Estrogen Antagonists

Tamoxifen has also been labeled with fluorine-18 for PET and radioactive iodine for single photon emission computed tomography (SPECT) imaging.[59] In a pilot PET study using [18F]fluorotamoxifen in 10 women with ER-positive breast tumors,[60] 2 out of 3 lesions were identified as true negative and 16 out of 20 lesions as true positive. Another pilot study with 9 patients has been conducted with [123I]iodotamoxifen in SPECT imaging. Tumor visualization was successful in 4 out of 6 patients with untreated breast carcinoma who had positive ER and PR expression.[61] The tumors that had both negative ER and PR expression or the tumors that had only expression of ER but not PR had no tracer uptake.

Fulvestrant, another endocrine drug, has been recently labeled at the 16α position with fluorine-18 for PET imaging.[62] However, because the binding affinity of the compound was greatly reduced by the addition of a fluorine atom at the 16α position, this tracer is unsuitable for PET imaging.

HER2/NEU

The HER2/neu status of a patient with breast cancer is measured by immunohistochemistry and fluorescence in situ hybridization, and this predicts response to HER2/neu targeted therapy, notably by trastuzumab.[63] However, as trastuzumab is now commonly used in the adjuvant setting, the role of HER2/neu targeted therapy at relapse is less clear. With several small-molecule drugs in development, the assessment of HER2/neu status in recurrent or metastatic sites is likely to become important. It has recently been shown that in patients receiving neoadjuvant chemotherapy plus trastuzumab, one-third of patients who fail to achieve a pathologic CR have lost HER2/neu expression during the course of treatment.[64] It has also been shown that differences can occur between the primary site and bone metastases.[65]

In a recent study, it has been shown that in vivo imaging of human epidermal factor receptor type 2 (HER 2) expression may allow direct assessment of HER2 status in tumor tissue and provide a means to quantify changes in receptor expression after HER2-targeted therapies. Affibody molecules are small and robust high-affinity protein molecules that can be engineered to bind specifically to a large number of target proteins. Results suggest that the described [18F-FBEM-Z HER2:342 affibody molecule can be used to assess HER2 expression in vivo by PET, and monitor possible changes of receptor expression in response to therapeutic interventions.[66,67]

Several investigators have radiolabeled trastuzumab, a monoclonal antibody constituting the current treatment of choice for HER2/neu positive breast cancer, with various isotopes, including [86]Y, ^{111}In, ^{90}Y, [76]Br, [203]Pb, ^{131}I, ^{99m}Tc, ^{68}Ga, and [64]Cu.[68–77] A recent study aimed to develop clinical-grade radiolabeled trastuzumab for clinical HER2/neu immunoPET scintigraphy, to improve diagnostic imaging, guide antibody-based therapy, and support early antibody development.[69] The antihuman epidermal growth factor receptor 2 (HER2/neu) antibody trastuzumab was administered to patients with HER2/neu-overexpressing breast cancer. HER2/neu scintigraphy helped to assess and quantify the HER2/neu expression of all lesions, including nonaccessible metastases. The study concluded that clinical grade [89]Zr-trastuzumab showed high and HER2/neu-specific tumor uptake at a good resolution.

PEPTIDE RECEPTORS

Peptides are attractive compounds for radiolabeling. Their typical small size, predominantly urinary excretion, and ease of synthesis and radiolabeling are favorable characteristics for imaging. Radiolabeled somatostatin was introduced several years ago to image somatostatin receptor expression in neuroendocrine tumors, first with radioiodinated analogues and later with radiolabeled [111In]pentetreotide, which remains the prime example of a successful tumor-imaging peptide.[78] Because of the high contrast achieved with neuroendocrine tumors, several groups have looked at somatostatin and other peptide receptors overexpressed in breast cancers as potential targets for imaging.

Somatostatin Receptors

Somatostatin receptors (SSTR) are present in several tissues such as the brain, pituitary, pancreas, and gastrointestinal tract. Various tumors have been reported to overexpress somatostatin receptors, including carcinoids, islet cell tumors, small cell lung cancers, pheochromocytomas, meningiomas, neuroblastomas, lymphomas (low density), renal cell tumors (low density), and hepatocellular carcinomas.[79] The overexpression of somatostatin receptors has been clearly demonstrated in breast cancers.[80–83] A clear positive correlation has been made between steroid hormone receptor expression and SSTR expression.[84] SSTR subtype 2 (SSTR2) expression was shown to correlate with ER and PR expression.[85,86] SSTR2 expression was also linked to lower tumor grade and longer survival in breast cancer patients.[80,85] Estrogen has been shown to influence SSTR2 expression, and the human sstr2 promoter area contains an estrogen response element.[87] Thus, there is a potential link between the estrogen responsiveness of a breast cancer and SSTR2 overexpression.

Many studies have demonstrated SSTR mRNA expression of various subtypes in most breast cancers.[81,83] mRNA levels have been shown to correlate relatively well with receptor protein expression in most breast cancers.[81] The primary use of SSTR imaging in the clinic is to characterize and stage neuroendocrine tumors. At present, several radiolabeled somatostatin analogues are available for scintigraphic imaging of the SSTR2.[88] Two somatostatin-derived tracers are generally available for planar and SPECT imaging: the radiolabeled cyclic peptides [^{111}In]DTPA-D-Phe1-octreotide ([^{111}In]pentetreotide or OctreoScan; Mallinckrodt) and [^{99m}Tc]depreotide (NeoSpect; Amersham). Each of these tracers has its own advantages: [^{111}In]pentetreotide provides better tumor to background ratios; [^{99m}Tc]depreotide benefits from the superior imaging characteristics of ^{99m}Tc. Other SSTR imaging radiopharmaceuticals, such as ^{99m}Tc-[HYNIC,Tyr^3]octreotide (^{99m}Tc-TOC) and ^{99m}Tc-[HYNIC,Tyr^3,Thr^8]octreotide (^{99m}Tc-TATE), are also available in some centers for research use.[89] Despite early enthusiasm, clinical results using radiolabeled somatostatin analogues for the diagnosis and staging of breast cancer have been largely disappointing. Van Eijck and colleagues[90] reported positive [^{111}In] DTPA-D-Phe1-octreotide scans in 39 of 52 primary breast cancers. Wang and colleagues[91] recently reported in a series of 55 cases a very high sensitivity with [^{99m}Tc]octreotide acetate (91.8%), but with a very poor specificity (22.2%). In a prospective study, Albérini and colleagues[92] detected only 4 of 11 malignant breast tumors with [^{111}In]-pentetreotide, despite the fact that 6 tumors expressed somatostatin receptors in vitro. These investigators concluded that somatostatin receptor scintigraphy was not sufficiently sensitive to detect primary breast tumors or axillary metastases.

The estrogen responsiveness of SSTR2 expression was examined with [^{99m}Tc]depreotide in breast cancer cell lines.[86] The findings indicate that estrogen-mediated response on SSTR2 expression could be monitored with [^{99m}Tc]depreotide SPECT. An important study by Van Den Bossche and colleagues[93] demonstrated the estrogen-dependent regulation of SSTR2 expression in patients with advanced breast cancer, using SPECT or planar scintigraphy with [^{99m}Tc]depreotide. Although sequential [^{99m}Tc]depreotide scintigraphy could predict therapy responsiveness with an accuracy of 100%, these results need to be validated by further research. **Fig. 2** illustrates a patient with metastatic breast cancer with positive [^{99m}Tc]depreotide scintigraphy who achieved prolonged disease stabilization with tamoxifen.

The development of PET tracers for SSTR2 will provide a significant improvement in diagnostic performance of nuclear imaging, due to intrinsic characteristics of PET that are superior to SPECT, such as improved spatial resolution, noise reduction, and attenuation correction. At present there are no PET tracers for SSTR2 that are routinely used in the clinic, but research in this area gives promising results. The new developments include labeling octreotide derivatives with fluorine-18 or gallium-68.

Gastrin-Releasing Peptide

Gastrin-releasing peptide (GRP) is a peptide that, in addition to its physiologic effects, has been implicated in the regulation of cell growth in some malignant cell lines.[94,95] A significant proportion of breast cancers express gastrin-releasing peptide receptors (GRPR).[96–99] The level of GRPR has been correlated positively with the presence of steroid hormone receptors in one study.[97] Bombesin (BBN), a potent GRPR ligand peptide, was first described by Anastasi and colleagues.[100]

Several investigators have successfully labeled derivatives of the active portion of BBN, notably with ^{111}In[101] as well as with ^{177}Lu, ^{99m}Tc, and ^{188}Re derivatives.[102–110] For PET imaging, Schuhmacher and colleagues[111] labeled a DOTA-PEG$_2$-[D-Tyr^6,β-Ala^{11},Thi^{13},Nle^{14}]BBN(6–14) with ^{68}Ga and ^{64}Cu,[112,113] whereas others have successfully labeled this peptide with ^{18}F.[114,115]

Few clinical results have been reported with radiolabelled bombesin analogues. Van de Wiele and colleagues[116] observed uptake of ^{99m}Tc-RP527, a bombesin analogue, in 4 of 6 patients with breast cancer, and were able to visualize bone metastases. Scopinaro and colleagues[117] reported visualization of 5 of 5 breast cancers with prone scintimammography using a [^{99m}Tc]bombesin peptide, with no

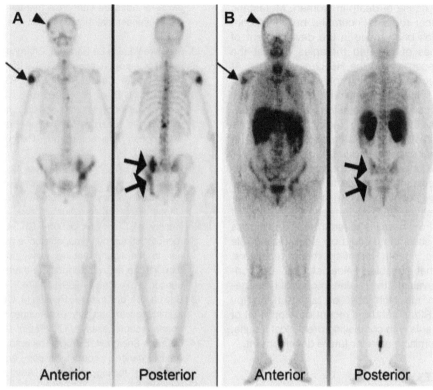

Fig. 2. A 57-year-old woman with metastatic breast cancer on bone scintigraphy (*A*). The bone metastases (*arrows*) expressed somatostatin receptors, as demonstrated with [99mTc]depreotide scintigraphy (*B*). (*From* Van Den Bossche B, Van Belle S, De Winter F, et al. Early prediction of endocrine therapy effect in advanced breast cancer patients using 99mTc-depreotide scintigraphy. J Nucl Med 2006;47:6–13; with permission from Society of Nuclear Medicine.)

undesirable side effects. This group reported visualization of 12 of 12 patients in an abstract published later, comparing [99mTc]bombesin with [99mTc]sestamibi scintimammography.[118]

Neuropeptide Y

Neuropeptide Y (NPY) is a 36–amino acid peptide involved in feeding behavior, anxiety, memory, and blood pressure regulation.[119] Reubi and colleagues[120,121] have shown a significant overexpression of NPY1R in 58% (45/77) to 85% (76/89) of breast tumors. Among these, 10 of 12 lobular carcinomas expressed NPY1R. Amlal and colleagues[122] found NPY1R on the MCF-7 human breast cancer cell line, and demonstrated that NPY1R expression was upregulated by estrogen. NPY inhibited the estrogen-induced cell proliferation. Langer and colleagues[123] successfully labeled modified NPY analogues with 99mTc for potential use in diagnostic imaging using 2-picolylamine-*N,N*-diacetic acid as a chelating agent, and obtained stable compounds with either nonselective (Y1 and Y2 binding) or selective Y2

binding. However, so far no clinical studies have been conducted with radiolabeled NPY ligands.

TRIPLE-NEGATIVE BREAST CANCER

Triple-negative (ER-negative/PR-negative/HER2-negative) breast carcinoma is a subclass of biologically more aggressive breast cancer.[124] In a recent study with 88 patients with breast cancer (29 patients are triple-negative), Basu and colleagues[125] found a sensitivity of 100% in this tumor subtype and higher [18F]FDG uptake compared with the ER-positive/PR-positive/HER2-negative breast tumors. Thus, in this group of patients [18F]FDG seems to perform very well due to high glucose uptake in this aggressive malignancy.

SUMMARY

Despite improvements in early diagnosis with the use of screening programs that lead to a high cure rate, breast cancer remains unfortunately a common cause of death in women. Metastatic breast cancer remains incurable, but significant progress has been made in the development of multiple lines of targeted therapies against the estrogen receptor and the HER2/neu protein. At present, receptor imaging plays no significant role in the clinical management of patients with primary, recurrent, or metastatic breast cancer, despite several promising radiopharmaceuticals that can directly image the targets of interest. It is hoped that ongoing and future clinical trials will provide guidance on how these tools are to be used in predicting response to targeted therapy. Given the high conversion rate of malignancies expressing either steroid hormone receptors or HER2/neu from baseline to recurrence and across metastatic sites, there could be a compelling role for imaging agents targeting these receptors, provided that suitable clinical studies are conducted to evaluate their value in clinical management. With the high cost of targeted therapy against HER2/neu and the recent development of imaging agents with compelling preclinical results, this is a promising area for future development.

REFERENCES

1. Brenton JD, Carey LA, Ahmed AA, et al. Molecular classification and molecular forecasting of breast cancer: ready for clinical application? J Clin Oncol 2005;23:7350.
2. Sorlie T, Perou CM, Tibshirani R, et al. Gene expression patterns of breast carcinomas distinguish tumor subclasses with clinical implications. Proc Natl Acad Sci U S A 2001;98:10869.
3. Ali S, Coombes RC. Endocrine-responsive breast cancer and strategies for combating resistance. Nat Rev Cancer 2002;2:101.
4. Winer EP, Hudis C, Burstein HJ, et al. American Society of Clinical Oncology technology assessment on the use of aromatase inhibitors as adjuvant therapy for postmenopausal women with hormone receptor-positive breast cancer: status report 2004. J Clin Oncol 2005;23:619 [see comment].
5. Agrup M, Stal O, Olsen K, et al. C-erbB-2 overexpression and survival in early onset breast cancer. Breast Cancer Res Treat 2000;63:23.
6. Piccart-Gebhart MJ, Procter M, Leyland-Jones B, et al. Trastuzumab after adjuvant chemotherapy in HER2-positive breast cancer. N Engl J Med 2005; 353:1659 [see comment].
7. Rakha EA, Reis-Filho JS, Ellis IO. Basal-like breast cancer: a critical review. J Clin Oncol 2008;26: 2568.
8. Bardou VJ, Arpino G, Elledge RM, et al. Progesterone receptor status significantly improves outcome prediction over estrogen receptor status alone for adjuvant endocrine therapy in two large breast cancer databases. J Clin Oncol 2003;21: 1973.
9. McGuire WL, De La Garza M, Chamness GC. Evaluation of estrogen receptor assays in human breast cancer tissue. Cancer Res 1977;37:637.
10. Leclercq G, Bojar H, Goussard J, et al. Abbott monoclonal enzyme immunoassay measurement of estrogen receptors in human breast cancer: a European multicenter study. Cancer Res 1986; 46:4233s.
11. DeSombre ER, Thorpe SM, Rose C, et al. Prognostic usefulness of estrogen receptor immunocytochemical assays for human breast cancer. Cancer Res 1986;46:4256s.
12. Harvey JM, Clark GM, Osborne CK, et al. Estrogen receptor status by immunohistochemistry is superior to the ligand-binding assay for predicting response to adjuvant endocrine therapy in breast cancer. J Clin Oncol 1999;17:1474.
13. Bosman FT, de Goeij AF, Rousch M. Quality control in immunocytochemistry: experiences with the oestrogen receptor assay. J Clin Pathol 1992;45:120.
14. Diaz LK, Sneige N. Estrogen receptor analysis for breast cancer: current issues and keys to increasing testing accuracy. Adv Anat Pathol 2005;12:10.
15. Hospers GA, Helmond FA, de Vries EG, et al. PET imaging of steroid receptor expression in breast and prostate cancer. Curr Pharm Des 2008;14: 3020.
16. Johnston SR, Saccani-Jotti G, Smith IE, et al. Changes in estrogen receptor, progesterone receptor, and pS2 expression in tamoxifen-resistant human breast cancer. Cancer Res 1995;55:3331.
17. Castagnetta L, Traina A, DiCarlo A, et al. Heterogeneity of soluble and nuclear oestrogen receptor status of involved nodes in relation to primary breast cancer. Eur J Cancer Clin Oncol 1987;23:31.
18. Webster DJ, Bronn DG, Minton JP. Estrogen receptor levels in multiple biopsies from patients with breast cancer. Am J Surg 1978;136:337.
19. Lee YT. Variability of steroid receptors in multiple biopsies of breast cancer: effect of systemic therapy. Breast Cancer Res Treat 1982;2:185.
20. Spataro V, Price K, Goldhirsch A, et al. Sequential estrogen receptor determinations from primary breast cancer and at relapse: prognostic and therapeutic relevance. The International Breast Cancer Study Group (formerly Ludwig Group). Ann Oncol 1992;3:733.
21. Dehdashti F, Mortimer JE, Siegel BA, et al. Positron tomographic assessment of estrogen receptors in breast cancer: comparison with FDG-PET and in vitro receptor assays. J Nucl Med 1995;36:1766.
22. Mankoff DA, Peterson LM, Petra PH, et al. Factors affecting the level and heterogeneity of uptake of

[18F]fluoroestradiol in patients with estrogen receptor positive breast cancer [abstract]. J Nucl Med 2002;43:286P.

23. McGuire AH, Dehdashti F, Siegel BA, et al. Positron tomographic assessment of 16 alpha-[18F] fluoro-17 beta-estradiol uptake in metastatic breast carcinoma. J Nucl Med 1991;32:1526.

24. Beauregard J, Turcotte E, Bénard F. Steroid receptor imaging in breast cancer. PET Clin 2006;1:51.

25. Hochberg RB. Iodine-125-labeled estradiol: a gamma-emitting analog of estradiol that binds to the estrogen receptor. Science 1979;205:1138.

26. Schober O, Scheidhauer K, Jackisch C, et al. Breast cancer imaging with radioiodinated oestradiol. Lancet 1990;335:1522.

27. Scheidhauer K, Muller S, Smolarz K, et al. Tumor-Szintigraphie mit 123J-markiertem Ostradiol beim Mammakarzinom-Rezeptorszintigraphie [Tumor scintigraphy using 123I-labeled estradiol in breast cancer receptor scintigraphy]. Nucl Med (Stuttg) 1991;30:84 [in German].

28. Ali H, Rousseau J, Gantchev TG, et al. 2- and 4-fluorinated 16 alpha[125I]iodoestradiol derivatives: synthesis and effect on estrogen receptor binding and receptor-mediated target tissue uptake. J Med Chem 1993;36:4255.

29. Ali H, Rousseau J, Paquette B, et al. Synthesis and biological properties of 7alpha-cyano derivatives of the (17alpha,20E/Z)-[125I]iodovinyl- and 16alpha-[125I]iodo-estradiols. Steroids 2003;68:1189.

30. Ali H, Rousseau J, van Lier JE. 7 alpha-Methyl- and 11 beta-ethoxy-substitution of [125I]-16 alpha-iodoestradiol: effect on estrogen receptor-mediated target tissue uptake. J Med Chem 1993;36:264.

31. Ali H, Rousseau J, van Lier JE. Synthesis of A-ring fluorinated derivatives of (17 alpha,20E/Z)-[125I]iodovinylestradiols: effect on receptor binding and receptor-mediated target tissue uptake. J Med Chem 1993;36:3061.

32. Foulon C, Guilloteau D, Baulieu JL, et al. Estrogen receptor imaging with 17 alpha-[123I]iodovinyl-11 beta-methoxyestradiol (MIVE2)—part I. Radiotracer preparation and characterization. Nuclear Medicine & Biology. Int J Rad Appl Instrum B 1992;19:257.

33. Nachar O, Rousseau JA, Lefebvre B, et al. Biodistribution, dosimetry and metabolism of 11beta-methoxy-(17alpha,20E/Z)-[123I]iodovinylestradiol in healthy women and breast cancer patients. J Nucl Med 1999;40:1728.

34. Nachar O, Rousseau JA, Ouellet R, et al. Scintimammography with 11beta-methoxy-(17alpha,20Z)-[123I]iodovinylestradiol: a complementary role to 99mTc-methoxyisobutyl isonitrile in the characterization of breast tumors. J Nucl Med 2000;41:1324.

35. Ribeiro-Barras MJ, Foulon C, Baulieu JL, et al. Estrogen receptor imaging with 17 alpha-[123I]iodovinyl-11 beta-methoxyestradiol (MIVE2)—part II. Preliminary results in patients with breast carcinoma. Nuclear Medicine & Biology. Int J Rad Appl Instrum B 1992;19:263.

36. Rijks LJ, Boer GJ, Endert E, et al. The Z-isomer of 11 beta-methoxy-17 alpha-[123I]iodovinylestradiol is a promising radioligand for estrogen receptor imaging in human breast cancer. Nucl Med Biol 1997;24:65.

37. Kiesewetter D, Kilbourn M, Landvatter S, et al. Preparation of four fluorine-18-labeled estrogens and their selective uptake in target tissues of immature rats. J Nucl Med 1984;25:1212.

38. Peterson LM, Mankoff DA, Lawton T, et al. Quantitative imaging of estrogen receptor expression in breast cancer with PET and 18F-fluoroestradiol. J Nucl Med 2008;49:367.

39. Tewson TJ, Mankoff DA, Peterson LM, et al. Interactions of 16alpha-[18F]-fluoroestradiol (FES) with sex steroid binding protein (SBP). Nucl Med Biol 1999;26:905.

40. Jonson SD, Bonasera TA, Dehdashti F, et al. Comparative breast tumor imaging and comparative in vitro metabolism of 16alpha-[18F]fluoroestradiol-17beta and 16beta-[18F]fluoromoxestrol in isolated hepatocytes. Nucl Med Biol 1999;26:123.

41. Mankoff DA, Peterson LM, Tewson TJ, et al. [18F]fluoroestradiol radiation dosimetry in human PET studies. J Nucl Med 2001;42:679.

42. Katzenellenbogen JA, Mathias CJ, VanBrocklin HF, et al. Titration of the in vivo uptake of 16 alpha-[18F]fluoroestradiol by target tissues in the rat: competition by tamoxifen, and implications for quantitating estrogen receptors in vivo and the use of animal models in receptor-binding radiopharmaceutical development. Nucl Med Biol 1993;20:735.

43. Yoo J, Dence CS, Sharp TL, et al. Synthesis of an estrogen receptor beta-selective radioligand: 5-[18F]fluoro-(2R,3S)-2,3-bis(4-hydroxyphenyl)pentanenitrile and comparison of in vivo distribution with 16alpha-[18F]fluoro-17beta-estradiol. J Med Chem 2005;48:6366.

44. VanBrocklin HF, Rocque PA, Lee HV, et al. 16 beta-[18F]fluoromoxestrol: a potent, metabolically stable positron emission tomography imaging agent for estrogen receptor positive human breast tumors. Life Sci 1993;53:811.

45. Bénard F, Aliaga A, Ahmed N, et al. Biodistribution of fluorinated estradiol derivatives in ER+ tumor-bearing mice: impact of substituents, formulation and specific activity. J Nucl Med 2004;45:329P [abstract].

46. Seimbille Y, Rousseau J, Benard F, et al. 18F-labeled difluoroestradiols: preparation and preclinical evaluation as estrogen receptor-binding radiopharmaceuticals. Steroids 2002;67:765.

47. Beauregard JM, Croteau E, Ahmed N, et al. Assessment of human biodistribution and dosimetry of 4-fluoro-11beta-methoxy-16alpha-^{18}F-fluoroestradiol using serial whole-body PET/CT. J Nucl Med 2009;50:100.

48. Lim JL, Zheng L, Berridge MS, et al. The use of 3-methoxymethyl-16 beta, 17 beta-epiestriol-O-cyclic sulfone as the precursor in the synthesis of F-18 16 alpha-fluoroestradiol. Nucl Med Biol 1996;23:911.

49. Mintun MA, Welch MJ, Siegel BA, et al. Breast cancer: PET imaging of estrogen receptors. Radiology 1988;169:45.

50. Mortimer JE, Dehdashti F, Siegel BA, et al. Positron emission tomography with 2-^{18}F]fluoro-2-deoxy-D-glucose and 16alpha-^{18}F]fluoro-17beta-estradiol in breast cancer: correlation with estrogen receptor status and response to systemic therapy. Clin Cancer Res 1996;2:933.

51. Mortimer JE, Dehdashti F, Siegel BA, et al. Metabolic flare: indicator of hormone responsiveness in advanced breast cancer. J Clin Oncol 2001;19:2797.

52. Dehdashti F, Mortimer JE, Trinkaus K, et al. PET-based estradiol challenge as a predictive biomarker of response to endocrine therapy in women with estrogen-receptor-positive breast cancer. Breast Cancer Res Treat 2009;113:509.

53. Linden HM, Stekhova SA, Link JM, et al. Quantitative fluoroestradiol positron emission tomography imaging predicts response to endocrine treatment in breast cancer. J Clin Oncol 2006;24:2793.

54. Verhagen A, Elsinga PH, de Groot TJ, et al. A fluorine-18 labeled progestin as an imaging agent for progestin receptor positive tumors with positron emission tomography. Cancer Res 1991;51:1930.

55. Dehdashti F, McGuire AH, Van Brocklin HF, et al. Assessment of 21-^{18}F]fluoro-16 alpha-ethyl-19-norprogesterone as a positron-emitting radiopharmaceutical for the detection of progestin receptors in human breast carcinomas. J Nucl Med 1991;32:1532.

56. Verhagen A, Studeny M, Luurtsema G, et al. Metabolism of a ^{18}F]fluorine labeled progestin (21-^{18}F]fluoro-16 alpha-ethyl-19-norprogesterone) in humans: a clue for future investigations. Nucl Med Biol 1994;21:941.

57. Vijaykumar D, Mao W, Kirschbaum KS, et al. An efficient route for the preparation of a 21-fluoro progestin-16 alpha,17 alpha-dioxolane, a high-affinity ligand for PET imaging of the progesterone receptor. J Org Chem 2002;67:4904.

58. Zhou D, Carlson KE, Katzenellenbogen JA, et al. Bromine- and iodine-substituted 16alpha,17alpha-dioxolane progestins for breast tumor imaging and radiotherapy: synthesis and receptor binding affinity. J Med Chem 2006;49:4737.

59. Yang DJ, Li C, Kuang LR, et al. Imaging, biodistribution and therapy potential of halogenated tamoxifen analogues. Life Sci 1994;55:53.

60. Inoue T, Kim EE, Wallace S, et al. Positron emission tomography using ^{18}F]fluorotamoxifen to evaluate therapeutic responses in patients with breast cancer: preliminary study. Cancer Biother Radiopharm 1996;11:235.

61. Van de Wiele C, Cocquyt V, VandenBroecke R, et al. Iodine-labeled tamoxifen uptake in primary human breast carcinoma. J Nucl Med 2001;42:1818.

62. Seimbille Y, Benard F, Rousseau J, et al. Impact on estrogen receptor binding and target tissue uptake of ^{18}F]fluorine substitution at the 16[alpha]-position of fulvestrant (faslodex; ICI 182,780). Nucl Med Biol 2004;31:691.

63. Carney WP, Leitzel K, Ali S, et al. HER-2/neu diagnostics in breast cancer. Breast Cancer Res 2007;9:207.

64. Mittendorf E, Esteva F, Wu Y, et al: Determination of HER2 status in patients achieving less than a pathologic complete response following neoadjuvant therapy with combination chemotherapy plus trastuzumab. In: ASCO 2008 Breast Cancer Symposium. Washington, DC, September 5–7, 2008.

65. Lorincz T, Toth J, Badalian G, et al. HER-2/neu genotype of breast cancer may change in bone metastasis. Pathol Oncol Res 2006;12:149.

66. Kramer-Marek G, Kiesewetter DO, Capala J. Changes in HER2 expression in breast cancer xenografts after therapy can be quantified using PET and (18)F-labeled affibody molecules. J Nucl Med 2009;50:1131.

67. Kramer-Marek G, Kiesewetter DO, Martiniova L, et al. [18]F]FBEM-Z(HER2:342)-Affibody molecule-a new molecular tracer for in vivo monitoring of HER2 expression by positron emission tomography. Eur J Nucl Med Mol Imaging 2008;35:1008.

68. Blend MJ, Stastny JJ, Swanson SM, et al. Labeling anti-HER2/neu monoclonal antibodies with ^{111}In and ^{90}Y using a bifunctional DTPA chelating agent. Cancer Biother Radiopharm 2003;18:355.

69. Dijkers EC, Kosterink JG, Rademaker AP, et al. Development and characterization of clinical-grade [89]Zr-trastuzumab for HER2/neu immunoPET imaging. J Nucl Med 2009;50:974.

70. Garmestani K, Milenic DE, Brady ED, et al. Purification of cyclotron-produced [203]Pb for labeling Herceptin. Nucl Med Biol 2005;32:301.

71. Garmestani K, Milenic DE, Plascjak PS, et al. A new and convenient method for purification of [86]Y using a Sr(II) selective resin and comparison of biodistribution of [86]Y and ^{111}In labeled Herceptin. Nucl Med Biol 2002;29:599.

72. Kobayashi H, Shirakawa K, Kawamoto S, et al. Rapid accumulation and internalization of radiolabeled

herceptin in an inflammatory breast cancer xeno-graft with vasculogenic mimicry predicted by the contrast-enhanced dynamic MRI with the macromolecular contrast agent G6-(1B4M-Gd)(256). Cancer Res 2002;62:860.

73. Lub-de Hooge MN, Kosterink JG, Perik PJ, et al. Preclinical characterisation of ^{111}In-DTPA-trastuzumab. Br J Pharmacol 2004;143:99.

74. Smith-Jones PM, Solit DB, Akhurst T, et al. Imaging the pharmacodynamics of HER2 degradation in response to Hsp90 inhibitors. Nat Biotechnol 2004;22:701 [see comment].

75. Tang Y, Scollard D, Chen P, et al. Imaging of HER2/neu expression in BT-474 human breast cancer xenografts in athymic mice using [(99m)Tc]-HYNIC-trastuzumab (Herceptin) Fab fragments. Nucl Med Commun 2005;26:427.

76. Tang Y, Wang J, Scollard DA, et al. Imaging of HER2/neu-positive BT-474 human breast cancer xenografts in athymic mice using (111)In-trastuzumab (Herceptin) Fab fragments. Nucl Med Biol 2005;32:51.

77. Winberg KJ, Persson M, Malmstrom PU, et al. Radiobromination of anti-HER2/neu/ErbB-2 monoclonal antibody using the p-isothiocyanatobenzene derivative of the [76Br]undecahydro-bromo-7,8-dicarba-nido-undecaborate(1-) ion. Nucl Med Biol 2004;31:425.

78. Krenning E, Kwekkeboom D, Pauwels S, et al. Somatostatin receptor scintigraphy. In: Freeman L, editor. Nuclear medicine annual. New York: Raven Press; 1995. p. 1.

79. van der Lely AJ, de Herder WW, Krenning EP, et al. Octreoscan radioreceptor imaging. Endocrine 2003;20:307.

80. Foekens JA, Portengen H, van Putten WL, et al. Prognostic value of receptors for insulin-like growth factor 1, somatostatin, and epidermal growth factor in human breast cancer. Cancer Res 1989;49:7002.

81. Kumar U, Grigorakis SI, Watt HL, et al. Somatostatin receptors in primary human breast cancer: quantitative analysis of mRNA for subtypes 1-5 and correlation with receptor protein expression and tumor pathology. Breast Cancer Res Treat 2005;92:175.

82. Schaer JC, Waser B, Mengod G, et al. Somatostatin receptor subtypes sst1, sst2, sst3 and sst5 expression in human pituitary, gastroentero-pancreatic and mammary tumors: comparison of mRNA analysis with receptor autoradiography. Int J Cancer 1997;70:530.

83. Schulz S, Schmitt J, Wiborny D, et al. Immunocytochemical detection of somatostatin receptors sst1, sst2A, sst2B, and sst3 in paraffin-embedded breast cancer tissue using subtype-specific antibodies. Clin Cancer Res 1998;4:2047.

84. Reubi JC, Torhorst J. The relationship between somatostatin, epidermal growth factor, and steroid hormone receptors in breast cancer. Cancer 1989;64:1254.

85. Pilichowska M, Kimura N, Suzuki A, et al. Clinico-pathological value of somatostatin type 2A and estrogen receptor immunoreactivity in human breast carcinoma. Endocr Pathol 2001;12:55.

86. Van Den Bossche B, D'Haeninck E, De Vos F, et al. Oestrogen-mediated regulation of somatostatin receptor expression in human breast cancer cell lines assessed with ^{99m}Tc-depreotide. Eur J Nucl Med & Mol Imaging 2004;31:1022.

87. Xu Y, Song J, Berelowitz M, et al. Estrogen regulates somatostatin receptor subtype 2 messenger ribonucleic acid expression in human breast cancer cells. Endocrinology 1996;137:5634.

88. Virgolini I, Traub T, Novotny C, et al. Experience with indium-111 and yttrium-90-labeled somatostatin analogs. Curr Pharm Des 2002;8:1781.

89. Cwikla JB, Mikolajczak R, Pawlak D, et al. Initial direct comparison of ^{99m}Tc-TOC and ^{99m}Tc-TATE in identifying sites of disease in patients with proven GEP NETs. J Nucl Med 2008;49:1060.

90. van Eijck CH, Krenning EP, Bootsma A, et al. Somatostatin-receptor scintigraphy in primary breast cancer. Lancet 1994;343:640 [see comment].

91. Wang F, Wang Z, Wu J, et al. The role of technetium-99m-labeled octreotide acetate scintigraphy in suspected breast cancer and correlates with expression of SSTR. Nucl Med Biol 2008;35:665.

92. Alberini JL, Meunier B, Denzler B, et al. Somatostatin receptor in breast cancer and axillary nodes: study with scintigraphy, histopathology and receptor autoradiography. Breast Cancer Res Treat 2000;61:21.

93. Van Den Bossche B, Van Belle S, De Winter F, et al. Early prediction of endocrine therapy effect in advanced breast cancer patients using ^{99m}Tc-depreotide scintigraphy. J Nucl Med 2006;47:6.

94. Mantey S, Frucht H, Coy DH, et al. Characterization of bombesin receptors using a novel, potent, radiolabeled antagonist that distinguishes bombesin receptor subtypes. Mol Pharmacol 1993;43:762.

95. Yegen BC. Bombesin-like peptides: candidates as diagnostic and therapeutic tools. Curr Pharm Des 2003;9:1013.

96. Gugger M, Reubi JC. Gastrin-releasing peptide receptors in non-neoplastic and neoplastic human breast. Am J Pathol 1999;155:2067.

97. Halmos G, Wittliff JL, Schally AV. Characterization of bombesin/gastrin-releasing peptide receptors in human breast cancer and their relationship to steroid receptor expression. Cancer Res 1995;55:280.

98. Pagani A, Papotti M, Sanfilippo B, et al. Expression of the gastrin-releasing peptide gene in carcinomas of the breast. Int J Cancer 1991;47:371.

99. Reubi JC, Wenger S, Schmuckli-Maurer J, et al. Bombesin receptor subtypes in human cancers: detection with the universal radioligand (125)I-[D-TYR(6), beta-ALA(11), PHE(13), NLE(14)] bombesin(6-14). Clin Cancer Res 2002;8:1139.

100. Anastasi A, Erspamer V, Bucci M. Isolation and structure of bombesin and alytesin, 2 analogous active peptides from the skin of the European amphibians Bombina and Alytes. Experientia 1971;27:166.

101. Hoffman TJ, Gali H, Smith CJ, et al. Novel series of ^{111}In-labeled bombesin analogs as potential radiopharmaceuticals for specific targeting of gastrin-releasing peptide receptors expressed on human prostate cancer cells. J Nucl Med 2003;44:823.

102. Ferro-Flores G, Arteaga de Murphy C, Rodriguez-Cortes J, et al. Preparation and evaluation of ^{99m}Tc-EDDA/HYNIC-[Lys 3]-bombesin for imaging gastrin-releasing peptide receptor-positive tumours. Nucl Med Commun 2006;27:371.

103. Gourni E, Paravatou M, Bouziotis P, et al. Evaluation of a series of new ^{99m}Tc-labeled bombesin-like peptides for early cancer detection. Anticancer Res 2006;26:435.

104. Johnson CV, Shelton T, Smith CJ, et al. Evaluation of combined (177)Lu-DOTA-8-AOC-BBN (7-14)NH(2) GRP receptor-targeted radiotherapy and chemotherapy in PC-3 human prostate tumor cell xenografted SCID mice. Cancer Biother Radiopharm 2006;21:155.

105. Lantry LE, Cappelletti E, Maddalena ME, et al. ^{177}Lu-AMBA: synthesis and characterization of a selective ^{177}Lu-labeled GRP-R agonist for systemic radiotherapy of prostate cancer. J Nucl Med 2006;47:1144.

106. Lin K-S, Luu A, Baidoo KE, et al. A new high affinity technetium-99m-bombesin analogue with low abdominal accumulation. Bioconjug Chem 2005;16:43.

107. Moustapha ME, Ehrhardt GJ, Smith CJ, et al. Preparation of cyclotron-produced [186]Re and comparison with reactor-produced [186]Re and generator-produced [188]Re for the labeling of bombesin. Nucl Med Biol 2006;33:81.

108. Smith CJ, Gali H, Sieckman GL, et al. Radiochemical investigations of ^{177}Lu-DOTA-8-Aoc-BBN[7-14]NH2: an in vitro/in vivo assessment of the targeting ability of this new radiopharmaceutical for PC-3 human prostate cancer cells. Nucl Med Biol 2003;30:101.

109. Smith CJ, Sieckman GL, Owen NK, et al. Radiochemical investigations of gastrin-releasing peptide receptor-specific [(99m)Tc(X)(CO)3-Dpr-Ser-Ser-Ser-Gln-Trp-Ala-Val-Gly-His-Leu-Met-(NH2)] in PC-3, tumor-bearing, rodent models: syntheses, radiolabeling, and in vitro/in vivo studies where Dpr = 2,3-diaminopropionic acid and X = H2O or P(CH2OH)3. Cancer Res 2003;63:4082.

110. Smith CJ, Sieckman GL, Owen NK, et al. Radiochemical investigations of [[188]Re(H_2O)(CO)3-diaminopropionic acid-SSS-bombesin(7-14)NH2]: syntheses, radiolabeling and in vitro/in vivo GRP receptor targeting studies. Anticancer Res 2003;23:63.

111. Schuhmacher J, Zhang H, Doll J, et al. GRP receptor-targeted PET of a rat pancreas carcinoma xenograft in nude mice with a ^{68}Ga-labeled bombesin(6–14) analog. J Nucl Med 2005;46:691.

112. Chen X, Park R, Hou Y, et al. microPET and autoradiographic imaging of GRP receptor expression with ^{64}Cu-DOTA-[Lys3]bombesin in human prostate adenocarcinoma xenografts. J Nucl Med 2004;45:1390 [see comment].

113. Rogers BE, Bigott HM, McCarthy DW, et al. Micro-PET imaging of a gastrin-releasing peptide receptor-positive tumor in a mouse model of human prostate cancer using a ^{64}Cu-labeled bombesin analogue. Bioconjug Chem 2003;14:756.

114. Hohne A, Mu L, Honer M, et al. Synthesis, ^{18}F-labeling, and in vitro and in vivo studies of bombesin peptides modified with silicon-based building blocks. Bioconjug Chem 2008;19:1871.

115. Zhang X, Cai W, Cao F, et al. ^{18}F-labeled bombesin analogs for targeting GRP receptor-expressing prostate cancer. J Nucl Med 2006;47:492.

116. Van de Wiele C, Dumont F, Vanden Broecke R, et al. Technetium-99m RP527, a GRP analogue for visualisation of GRP receptor-expressing malignancies: a feasibility study. Eur J Nucl Med 2000;27:1694.

117. Scopinaro F, Varvarigou AD, Ussof W, et al. Technetium labeled bombesin-like peptide: preliminary report on breast cancer uptake in patients. Cancer Biother Radiopharm 2002;17:327.

118. Scopinaro F, De Vincentis G, Ussof W, et al. Prone scintimammography with 13Leu bombesin Tc-99m: comparison with sestamibi scintimammography. Eur J Nucl Med 2002;29:S68.

119. Inui A. Neuropeptide Y: a key molecule in anorexia and cachexia in wasting disorders? Mol Med Today 1999;5:79.

120. Reubi C, Gugger M, Waser B. Co-expressed peptide receptors in breast cancer as a molecular basis for in vivo multireceptor tumour targeting. Eur J Nucl Med Mol Imaging 2002;29:855.

121. Reubi JC, Gugger M, Waser B, et al. Y(1)-mediated effect of neuropeptide Y in cancer: breast carcinomas as targets. Cancer Res 2001;61:4636.

122. Amlal H, Faroqui S, Balasubramaniam A, et al. Estrogen up-regulates neuropeptide Y Y1 receptor expression in a human breast cancer cell line. Cancer Res 2006;66:3706.

123. Langer M, La Bella R, Garcia-Garayoa E, et al. ^{99m}Tc-labeled neuropeptide Y analogues as potential tumor imaging agents. Bioconjug Chem 2001;12:1028.

124. Haffty BG, Yang Q, Reiss M, et al. Locoregional relapse and distant metastasis in conservatively managed triple negative early-stage breast cancer. J Clin Oncol 2006;24:5652 [see comment].
125. Basu S, Chen W, Tchou J, et al. Comparison of triple-negative and estrogen receptor-positive/progesterone receptor-positive/HER2-negative breast carcinoma using quantitative fluorine-18 fluorodeoxyglucose/positron emission tomography imaging parameters: a potentially useful method for disease characterization. Cancer 2008;112:995.

Screening of Contralateral Breast in Patients with Breast Cancer: Role of MR Imaging and PET/CT Imaging

Susan Weinstein, MD[a], Madhavi Chawla, MD[b],
Rakesh Kumar, MD[b],*

KEYWORDS

- Contralateral breast screening
- Magentic resonance imaging
- PET • PET-CT • Breast cancer

Breast cancer is one of the most common cancers in women. Contralateral breast carcinoma is the most common second malignancy in patients with breast carcinoma, with an incidence as high as 12%.[1,2] Bilateral breast carcinomas exist in 2 forms, synchronous, in which both tumors occur at the same time, or metachronous, in which they occur at different times. The incidence of synchronous breast cancer, detected clinically, on imaging, or by both methods, is estimated to be approximately 1% to 7%.[3,4] When a woman is diagnosed with breast cancer, the contralateral breast should be carefully evaluated for a synchronous tumor. There are many reasons why screening for occult contralateral breast cancer is so important on initial cancer diagnosis (**Fig. 1**). The detection and treatment of a synchronous tumor allows for informed surgical decision making, especially if tissue reconstruction is being considered. Abdominal tissue flaps, such as the transverse rectus abdominis muscle flap, may be performed only once. If a second flap is needed at a later date, tissue will need to be harvested from elsewhere, such as the latissimus dorsi, or implant reconstruction would be the alternative. If

chemotherapy is necessary, the patient would only need treatment once for bilateral synchronous cancers, not twice, as would be the situation for metachronous cancers. Significant mortality is associated metachronous cancers in the contralateral breast; 7% being fatal.[5]

MAGNETIC RESONANCE IMAGING

There are multiple reports of magnetic resonance (MR) imaging-detected contralateral breast cancers in women, even in the setting of negative mammography and sonography. The incidence of cancers detected only by MR imaging is reported to be 3% to 24%.[6–12] MR imaging allows for early detection of synchronous contralateral breast cancer before the cancer becomes clinically evident, mammographically visible, or possibly when it is at an advanced stage.

One of the earliest published studies primarily addressing the detection of contralateral cancers by MR imaging alone was reported by Slanetz and colleagues[6] in 2002. Under an institutional review board-approved research protocol, 17 women with known breast cancers underwent

a Department of Radiology, Division of Breast Imaging, University of Pennsylvania Medical Center, 3400 Spruce Street, 1 Silverstein Building, Philadelphia, PA 19104, USA
b Department of Nuclear Medicine, All India Institute of Medical Sciences, New Delhi 110029, India
* Corresponding author.
E-mail address: rkphulia@hotmail.com (R. Kumar).

PET Clin 4 (2009) 343–347
doi:10.1016/j.cpet.2009.09.009
1556-8598/09/$ – see front matter © 2009 Published by Elsevier Inc.

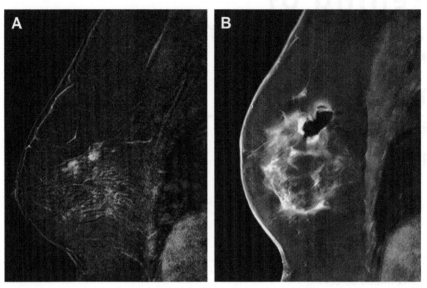

Fig. 1. 73-year-old woman recently diagnosed with left breast cancer. Mammography findings and clinical breast examination of the right breast were negative. Evaluation of the contralateral breast shows 2 enhancing masses in the superior breast (A). The patient underwent MR imaging-guided core needle biopsy (B). Pathology revealed invasive lobular carcinoma.

bilateral MR imaging examinations. Known cancer was identified in all 17 patients. In 5 of 17 patients, contralateral suspicious breast lesions were detected. In 4 of 5 patients, biopsy revealed invasive carcinoma that was clinically and mammographically occult , ranging in size from 6 mm to 5 cm. One patient had a fibroadenoma. The positive predictive value (PPV) of the MR imaging at the patient level was 24% (4 of 17).

Additional articles followed confirming MR imaging detection of mammographically and clinically occult contralateral breast cancer in patients who had been recently diagnosed with breast cancer. In a single institution retrospective study, Liberman and colleagues[8] analyzed 223 women who had contralateral MR imaging screening examinations. The patients enrolled in the study had negative results from mammograms and clinical breast examinations within 6 months of the MR imaging study. Twelve cancers were detected with a cancer detection rate of 5% (12 of 223). Six of them were invasive carcinomas and 6, ductal carcinoma in situ. The average size of the invasive carcinoma was 5 mm. The biopsy recommendation rate was 32% (72 of 223). Sixty-one women had the recommended biopsy, yielding a PPV of 20% (12 of 61).

The first multicenter prospective trial to address the contralateral MR imaging screening question was performed by the International Breast Magnetic Resonance Consortium (IBMC).[11] The 108 patients recruited for the study had a recent diagnosis of unilateral breast cancer and negative results from mammograms and clinical breast examinations within 90 days of the contralateral MR imaging screening. Five women were excluded, leaving 103 women in the final analysis. Biopsy was recommended in 12 of 103 women (12%) yielding 4 cancers. The PPV of an abnormal MR image was 4 of 12 (33%). The average size of the 4 cancers was 13.2 mm (range 8–17 mm).

The largest prospective contralateral MR imaging screening trial to date was sponsored by the American College of Radiology Imaging Network (ACRIN).[12] The final analysis included 969 women in whom 30 (3.1%) cancers that were mammographically and clinically occult were detected. Biopsy was performed in 12.5% (121) women with a PPV of 24.8% (30 of 121). There were 12 ductal carcinomas in situ and 18 invasive carcinomas. The average size of the invasive carcinoma was 10.9 mm. The sensitivity of mammography has been shown to be high in fatty breast, with decreasing sensitivity in the dense breast; because sensitivity of MR imaging is not affected by the breast density, one would expect to have a higher MR imaging screening detection rate in patients with dense breast tissue. However, the cancer detection rate in the study was not related to breast density or menopausal status.

PET AND PET-COMPUTED TOMOGRAPHY

PET with 2-[fluorine 18]fluoro-2-deoxy-D-glucose (FDG), being a technique based on increased uptake of radiolabelled glucose by tumor cells is useful in detection, staging, and restaging of a wide range of tumors, including breast cancer, and assessing response to therapy in them.[13–17] FDG PET may be helpful in detecting unsuspected contralateral breast tumor in patients with known breast cancer in the preoperative evaluation scan (synchronous) or in scans done later in the course of the disease (synchronous or metachronous).

FDG PET serves as a complementary imaging modality to MR imaging in detecting and characterizing locoregional breast cancer metastases. FDG PET being a whole body imaging modality, the contralateral breast is invariably screened when the ipsilateral breast with the known cancer is being evaluated (**Fig. 2**). Although FDG PET cannot resolve detailed axillary anatomy, it can clarify the nature of MR imaging abnormalities as metabolically active tumor versus scarring from previous treatment. FDG PET can also be used to identify sites of disease outside the suspected axillary recurrence. With the use of quantitative tissue characterization, PET can be used to detect the extent of disease with potentially more specific tumor identification than is possible with MR imaging and may reveal the presence of unsuspected metastases outside the axilla. Eubank and colleagues[18] found a sensitivity, specificity, and accuracy of 85%, 90%, and 88%, respectively, for FDG PET while staging mediastinal and intramammary lymph nodes in patients with metastatic breast cancer.

Whether bilateral breast cancers have an independent origin or are the result of a breast-to-breast metastasis may be crucial, because the therapeutic management of independent breast carcinoma is different from the treatment of metastatic disease.[19–21] The recently developed ability to acquire simultaneous PET and computed tomography (CT) scans allows the physiologic information obtained from the PET scan to be combined with high resolution, anatomic information provided by CT images. Also, PET-CT–guided biopsy can be performed, which targets the most metabolically active site, helping ascertain the histology of the tumor and thus, differentiate a second breast primary tumor from breast-to-breast metastasis. Combined FDG PET and MR imaging also provides useful treatment-planning data for patients clinically suspected of having recurrent axillary or supraclavicular breast cancer. Correlation of PET data with the anatomic information derived from MR imaging results in data that help to determine the approach to local and systemic therapy in patients suspected of having recurrent or advanced axillary disease.

There is high contrast between FDG uptake by tumors and that by most benign tissues; however, the limited spatial resolution[14] and artificially high metabolic activity in fat tissue, muscle, and bowel[22,23] hinders the use of FDG PET in detecting small tumors and prevents precise determination of the relationship of tumor masses to the chest wall and regional neurovascular structures. Fused PET-CT/visual combination of PET and CT have an advantage over morphologic and functional imaging procedures alone.[24,25]

The authors retrospectively analyzed the data of patients with known breast cancer referred for PET-CT for restaging at their department over a period of 1 year. A total of 234 patients of breast cancer underwent ^{18}F-FDG PET/CT over a period of 1 year for the purpose of staging/restaging. Bilateral breast cancers were found in 12 of 234 patients (5.1%). Synchronous tumors were found

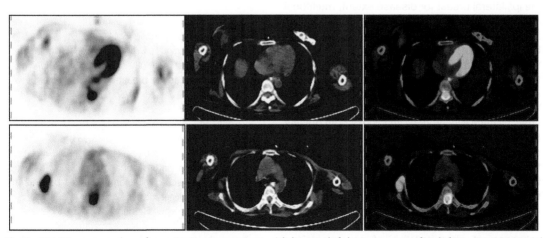

Fig. 2. PET-CT scan was done for restaging in a patient with known left breast cancer after left mastectomy. Axial sections of CT, PET, and PET-CT show metachronous nodular lesion on CT and focal area of abnormal uptake in the right breast on PET and PET-CT. Right axillary lymph nodes are also seen, suggestive of axillary metastasis.

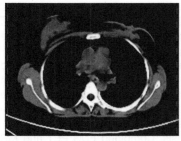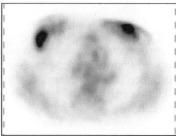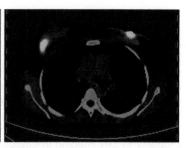

Fig. 3. Axial sections of CT, PET, and PET-CT showing synchronous focal areas of abnormal uptake in bilateral breasts. Due to bilateral dense breasts, CT findings may not suggest any pathology.

in 4 (33.3%) patients; whereas metachronous tumors were found in 8 patients (66.6%) **(Figs. 2 and 3)**. Increased FDG uptake was seen in all of these lesions. A suspicion of tumor was raised because of abnormal intense ^{18}F-FDG uptake in the other breast and was confirmed by further evaluation. Thus ^{18}F-FDG PET/CT detected tumor in the contralateral breast in 2.1% (5 of 234) of patients and accounted for 41.6% (5 of 12) of the bilateral breast tumors in this series.[26]

SUMMARY

Multiple studies over the years have demonstrated that contralateral MR imaging screening can detect mammographically and clinically occult breast cancer. The average size of the cancers in the IBMC study and the ACRIN contralateral screening trial was over 1 cm, which is not clinically insignificant. There are many reasons why MR imaging screening of the contralateral breast is advantageous. MR imaging evaluation of the ipsilateral is a well-accepted clinical indication in women with known breast cancer. MR imaging can evaluate the ipsilateral breast for disease extent, multifocal or multicentric carcinoma, and chest wall invasion. In the past, bilateral synchronous imaging of both breasts was not possible. If the contralateral breast needed to be imaged, it was necessary to subject the patient to 2 separate days of imaging, needing intravenous contrast to be administered twice. With advances in technology, using bilateral multicoil array, bilateral synchronous imaging of both breasts is possible. Therefore, the contralateral breast can easily be screened when the ipsilateral breast with the known cancer is being evaluated. In addition, the high spatial resolution of MR imaging makes morphologic evaluation possible. Additional information is obtained by rapid image acquisition that allows for assessment of kinetic information or enhancement characteristics of any suspicious lesions. Perhaps, the most important aspect of MR imaging contralateral screening is the ability to

target and biopsy any suspicious lesions that are detected.

Being a whole body imaging modality, FDG PET enables evaluation of the whole body during a single sitting, allowing the detection and characterization of primary breast cancer in contralateral breast and local-regional breast cancer metastases. Although FDG PET cannot resolve detailed axillary anatomy, it can clarify the nature of MR imaging abnormalities as metabolically active tumor versus scarring from previous treatment. PET and PET-CT have better specificity as compared with MRI, which has a higher sensitivity in detecting cancer in contralateral breast. Both studies can thus be used together to obtain a higher sensitivity and specificity in this clinical setting.

ACKNOWLEDGMENTS

This work also was supported in part by the Council of Scientific and Industrial Research, New Delhi, India under Senior Research Associate Fellowship.

REFERENCES

1. Pomerantz RA, Murad T, Hines JR. Bilareal breast cancer. Am Surg 1989;55:441–4.
2. Kurtz JM, Amalric R, Brandone H, et al. Contralateral breast cancer and other second malignancies in patients treated by breast-conserving therapy with radiation. Int J Radiat Oncol Biol Phys 1988;15: 277–84.
3. Egan RL. Bilateral breast carcinomas: Role of mammography. Cancer 1976;38:931.
4. Hungness ES, Safa M, Shaughnessy EA, et al. Bilateral synchronous breast cancer: mode of detection and comparison of histologic features between the 2 breasts. Surgery 2000;128:702.
5. Rosen PP, Groshen S, Kinne DW, et al. Contralateral breast carcinoma: an assessment of risk and prognosis in stage I (T1N0M0) and stage II (T1N1M0) patients with 20-year follow-up. Surgery 1989;106: 904.

6. Slanetz PJ, Edmister WB, Yeh ED, et al. Occult contralateral breast carcinoma incidentally detected by breast magnetic resonance imaging. Breast J 2002;8:145.

7. Pediconi F, Catalano C, Roselli A, et al. Contrast-enhanced MR mammography for evaluation of the contralateral breast in patients with diagnosed unilateral breast cancer or high-risk lesions. Radiology 2007;243:670.

8. Liberman L, Morris EA, Kim CM, et al. MR imaging findings in the contralateral breast of women with recently diagnosed breast cancer. AJR Am J Roentgenol 2003;180:333.

9. Lee SG, Orel SG, Woo IJ, et al. MR imaging screening of the contralateral breast in patients with newly diagnosed breast cancer: preliminary results. Radiology 2003;226:773.

10. Fischer U, Kopka L, Grabbe E. Breast carcinoma: effect of preoperative contrast-enhanced MR imaging on the therapeutic approach. Radiology 1999;213:881.

11. Lehman CD, Blume JD, Thickman D, et al. Added cancer yield of MRI in screening the contralateral breast of women recently diagnosed with breast cancer: results from the International Breast Magnetic Resonance Consortium (IBMC) trial. J Surg Oncol 2005;92:9.

12. Lehman CD, Gatsonis C, Kuhl CK, et al. MRI evaluation of the contralateral breast in women with recently diagnosed breast cancer. N Engl J Med 2007;356:1295.

13. Adler LP, Crowe JP, Al-Kaisi NK, et al. Evaluation of breast masses and axillary lymph nodes with [F-18] 2-deoxy-2- fluoro-D-glucose PET. Radiology 1993; 187:743–50.

14. Avril N, Dose J, Janicke F, et al. Assessment of axillary lymph node involvement in breast cancer patients with positron emission tomography using radiolabeled 2-(fluorine-18)-fluoro-2-deoxy-D-glucose. J Natl Cancer Inst 1996;88:1204–9.

15. Moon DH, Maddahi J, Silverman DHS, et al. Accuracy of whole-body fluorine-18- FDG PET for the detection of recurrent or metastatic breast carcinoma. J Nucl Med 1998;39:431–5.

16. Wahl RL, Zasadny K, Helvie M, et al. Metabolic monitoring of breast cancer chemohormonotherapy using positron emission tomography: initial evaluation. J Clin Oncol 1993;11:2101–11.

17. Bassa P, Kim EE, Inoue T, et al. Evaluation of preoperative chemotherapy using PET with fluorine-18-fluorodeoxyglucose in breast cancer. J Nucl Med 1996;37:931–8.

18. Eubank WB, Mankoff DA, Takasugi J, et al. 18fluorodeoxyglucose positron emission tomography to detect mediastinal or internal mammary metastases in breast cancer. J Clin Oncol 2001;19:3516–23.

19. Burns PE, Dabbs K, May C, et al. Bilateral breast cancer in northern Alberta: risk factors and survival patterns. Can Med Assoc J 1984;130: 881–6.

20. Dawson PJ, Maloney T, Gimotty P, et al. Bilateral breast cancer; one disease or two? Breast Cancer Res Treat 1991;19:233–44.

21. Coradini D, Oriana S, Mariani L, et al. Is steroid receptor profile in contralateral breast cancer a marker of independence of the corresponding primary tumor? Eur J Cancer 1998;34:825–30.

22. Yeung HW, Grewal RK, Gonen M, et al. Patterns of (18)F-FDG uptake in adipose tissue and muscle: a potential source of false-positives for PET. J Nucl Med 2003;44:1789–96.

23. Engel H, Steinert H, Buck A, et al. Whole-body PET: physiological and artifactual fluorodeoxyglucose accumulations. J Nucl Med 1996;37:441–6.

24. Antoch G, Saoudi N, Kuehl H, et al. Accuracy of whole-body dual-modality fluorine-18-2-fluoro-2-deoxy-D-glucose positron emission tomography and computed tomography (FDG-PET/CT) for tumor staging in solid tumors: comparison with CT and PET. J Clin Oncol 2004;22:4357–68.

25. Antoch G, Vogt FM, Freudenberg LS, et al. Whole-body dual-modality PET/CT and whole-body MRI for tumor staging in oncology. JAMA 2003;290: 3199–206.

26. Nadig MR, Kumar R, Patel CD, et al. Detection of contralateral breast cancer in patients with known breast cancer undergoing PET-CT scan for restaging. J Nucl Med 2007;48(Suppl):367 P (1572).

PET/CT in Radiation Therapy Planning for Breast Cancer

Sushil Beriwal, MD

KEYWORDS

- Functional imaging • ^{18}F fluorodeoxyglucose
- Metabolic FDG-PET imaging

Precise anatomic information regarding the location and extent of tumor tissue is essential for radiation treatment planning. Anatomic imaging has greatly improved the accuracy of delineating target structures and is currently the basis of modern 3-dimension (3D)-based radiation treatment.[1] Plain radiography, computed tomography (CT), and magnetic resonance (MR) imaging provide structural or morphologic information based on tissue density, size, vascularity, and fat or water content and are routinely being used for radiation treatment planning. The excellent spatial resolution of anatomic imaging techniques allows the detection of subcentimeter lesions (eg, in the lungs); however, definition of tumor involvement, for example in lymph nodes, based on the increased size is more difficult. Some enlarged lymph nodes may be reactive, whereas smaller nodes may harbor metastatic foci. MR imaging is better at outlining soft tissues, particularly in the brain, and has been valuable in complementing CT-based radiation treatment planning.[2]

Over recent years, functional imaging with PET has gained increased importance in determining biologic or molecular abnormalities in specific tumors. PET using ^{18}F fluorodeoxyglucose (FDG) allows the characterization of suspicious masses and the determination of the spread of disease to locoregional lymph nodes and distant sites.[3] The metabolic information derived from FDG-PET influences the radiation treatment planning in several ways. First, FDG-PET may reveal a tumor target that was previously not detected by anatomic imaging. Second, FDG-PET may detect additional tumor regions outside the tumor volume defined by CT or MR imaging. Third, FDG-PET may show subregions or foci with increased or altered biologic activity within the gross tumor volume that could be preferentially targeted and treated with escalated radiation doses. Therefore, the more precise 3D delineation of tumor volumes could translate into improved locoregional control with radiation therapy.

Breast cancer remains the most common nondermatologic cancer among women in the United States. In 2008, more than 250,000 new cases were expected to be diagnosed, including 184,000 cases of invasive disease and 68,000 cases of in situ (noninvasive) disease.[4] Breast irradiation was first used to minimize the risk of locoregional recurrence in patients who had locally advanced cancers.[5] Beginning in the late 1970s, breast irradiation has evolved into the mainstay of therapy in patients treated with breast conservation surgery. In recent years, breast conservation therapy consisting of a segmental mastectomy and definitive breast irradiation has assumed an increasing role in the management of patients who have invasive and noninvasive breast cancer. No fewer than 6 prospective, randomized controlled trials have shown equivalent outcomes of breast conservation therapy when compared with mastectomy.[6–11] Distant metastases of breast cancer are frequently found in lymph nodes, lungs, liver, and bones.

In the metastatic setting, radiation therapy is currently used for treatment of soft tissue and bone metastasis and also for intracranial disease.

Department of Radiation Oncology, University of Pittsburgh Cancer Institute, Magee-Womens Hospital of UPMC, 300 Halket Street, Pittsburgh, PA 15213, USA
E-mail address: beriwals@upmc.edu

PET Clin 4 (2009) 349–357
doi:10.1016/j.cpet.2009.09.007

Palliative radiation has been shown to be effective in improving the quality of life and providing relief of symptoms, especially the pain of bone metastasis.

For the last half century, breast irradiation has been performed through parallel opposing tangential beams with wedges with matching anterior supraclavicular and posterior axillary fields, whenever appropriate. Radiation simulation, the process of selecting the beam and the area to be treated, is routinely performed through fluoroscopic placement of the tangential beams based on clinically determined breast tissue borders. Treatment planning has been a single-slice, 2-dimensional (2D) dosimetry, applying wedge beam data onto manually obtained breast central axis contours.

Although this unsophisticated technique initially produced a breakthrough in breast conservation therapy, several significant limitations of this technique are now apparent including excess cardiac and lung sequelae of breast irradiation.[12] In addition, patients desire better cosmetic results and shorter treatment times. Increased scatter radiation to contralateral breast from wedges may increase the incidence of second malignant neoplasm.[13] Furthermore, some have suggested that poor dose distribution may contribute to late in-breast tumor failures. Data from Bhatnagar and colleagues[14] suggest significant reduction of scatter radiation to the contralateral breast with the use of intensity-modulated radiation therapy. As a result, newer techniques using CT-based treatment planning have been used to create "beam's eye" views to avoid these underlying critical structures.

CT-based 3D treatment planning represents an evolution from 2D planning and provides volumetric information that permits a greater assessment of the beam's path and subsequent dose to target tissues and normal structures. CT-based approaches also permit virtual simulation, a process in which the CT data set is acquired rapidly, thus significantly reducing the time the patient is spending on the simulation table. Treatment of chest wall and regional nodes poses significant challenges to radiation oncologists, particularly in the postmastectomy setting. The range of body habitus and close proximity of the internal mammary (IM) nodes to the heart often necessitates individualized treatment planning, with complex field arrangements. 3D treatment planning with volumetric information helps in clinical decision making.

CT-assisted volume definition remains the gold standard for planning external beam radiation therapy with curative intent.[1] Accurate localization of the gross tumor volume is critical to optimize the therapeutic ratio by sparing normal tissues and maximizing the coverage of tumor volumes in conformal radiation techniques. Use of currently available anatomic imaging for treatment planning has several limitations. These include the poor visualization and imprecise delineation of tumors in certain areas of the body (such as the head and neck) and the distorted anatomy postsurgically and in residual scar tissue after chemotherapy, specifically in previously irradiated areas. The incorporation of metabolic FDG-PET imaging in radiation treatment planning has raised hopes for further improvement, which would lead to so-called multidimensional conformal radiotherapy.

Breast cancer may be unique in that there are numerous locoregional treatments using various combinations of surgical techniques and radiotherapy regimens. Surgery may vary from lumpectomy, quadrantectomy, simple mastectomy, modified radical mastectomy, and even to radical mastectomy. There are several accepted radiation therapy techniques, ranging from treatment of the entire breast, with or without a boost to the lumpectomy cavity after breast conservation surgery, to more comprehensive techniques including the regional nodes.[15] These nodal areas include the axilla, supraclavicular region, and the upper IM region. Similarly, after the mastectomy, radiotherapy may be administered only to the chest wall or to the chest wall with 1 or more of the regional nodal areas.

There are important differences between the currently used anatomic imaging–based radiation treatment planning and the potential FDG-PET–based treatment planning. Although FDG-PET offers unique metabolic information about the tumor activity, the limited spatial resolution of PET compared with CT or MR imaging may not characterize small lesions with sufficient accuracy. Current PET technology does not allow the identification of micrometastases, which limits its use for narrowing the treatment volume in lymph node areas at risk. The specificity of FDG-PET is in the range from 80% to 95% and is generally higher than that of CT or MR imaging; however, the uptake of FDG is not specific for tumor tissue and granulomatous or acute inflammatory processes can result in false-positive PET findings. An important limitation of FDG-PET in radiation treatment planning is the imprecise delineation of tumor tissue based on the PET images. Unlike anatomic imaging, the size of metabolic abnormalities varies depending on the scaling of the PET display. Whereas tumors often have well-defined anatomic borders on CT images, the edges of tumors on FDG-PET imaging appear indistinct to the contouring physician. Some have arbitrarily defined the FDG-avid volume as the region encompassed by the 40% to 50%[16] intensity level relative to the tumor maximum, whereas others have normalized to the FDG uptake in the liver without background subtraction[17]; hence the FDG-avid volume may have significant interobserver variability. The use of standardized uptake value (SUV)-normalized parametric images may help to overcome this problem but again may miss necrotic tumor, which would have lower SUV uptake.

Following are the indications for which radiation therapy is used in breast cancer. Each is discussed in more detail later.

- Adjuvant radiation therapy after breast conserving surgery for all patients
- Adjuvant postmastectomy radiation therapy in a select subset of patients after mastectomy
- Radiation therapy for isolated locoregional recurrence after mastectomy
- Radiation therapy for metastatic disease.

ADJUVANT RADIATION THERAPY AFTER BREAST CONSERVING SURGERY FOR ALL PATIENTS

There is at present no role of PET/CT in radiation planning after breast conserving surgery. These patients are simulated with a custom-molded immobilization cradle or a breast board, which is created for each patient with the goal of ensuring consistent positioning during the treatment sessions. Radiopaque wires are taped to the skin to delineate the anatomic boundaries of the breast and the lumpectomy scar, and then CT simulation scans are obtained. The treatment fields are then designed on the CT simulation data set with the aid of treatment planning computers. The goal of field design is to include the targeted regions, which include the entire breast with lumpectomy cavity while avoiding normal structures such as the heart and lungs. The dimensions of the treatment fields are determined, and the optimal beam entrance angles are verified in the axial, coronal, and sagittal planes. Optimal beam arrangements for breast treatment typically consist of 2 opposing beams that tangentially cross the ipsilateral anterior thorax and minimize the volume of lung and heart in the field. The lumpectomy cavity as defined on CT receives an additional boost. There is a small study in the literature evaluating FDG-PET/CT to define lumpectomy cavity.[18] The targets defined using PET/CT were

significantly larger than those defined with CT alone; probably because of postoperative inflammatory changes in the cavity. These increased volumes could be covered by treatment plans with only a modest increase in irradiated tissue volume compared with CT-determined volumes. This study suggests difference in boost volumes, but in the absence of outcome data and excellent results with CT-based planning there is at present no role of PET/CT for radiation planning in this setting.

ADJUVANT POSTMASTECTOMY RADIATION THERAPY IN A SELECTED SUBSET OF PATIENTS AFTER MASTECTOMY

Three randomized trials have demonstrated an overall survival benefit with postmastectomy radiation in a selected subset of patients with breast cancer.[19–21] In these trials, patients were treated with comprehensive chest wall radiation, which included a supraclavicular field and IM field. The clinical practice guidelines of the American Society of Clinical Oncology recommend postmastectomy radiation in patients with 4 or more involved lymph nodes.[21] The panel recommended a supraclavicular field in patients with 4 or more involved axillary lymph nodes because of the risk of clinical failure in the region, but there was insufficient evidence to make suggestions or recommendations on whether deliberate IM nodal irradiation should or should not be used in any patient subgroup. The results of studies by the European Organisation for Research and Treatment of Cancer and the National Cancer Institute of Canada that randomized patients to receive or not receive supraclavicular and IM nodal radiation would help in some clarification of this issue. Thus routine use of radiation to treat the IM lymph nodes in women who have locally advanced breast cancer remains controversial; however, IM disease has been associated with higher rates of distant metastases and lower overall survival.[22] Although older extended radical mastectomy series did not demonstrate a survival advantage to IM dissection, they did demonstrate that for medially located tumors the incidence of involvement was up to 40%, especially when the axilla was also positive for metastases.[23,24] In subset analyses, there was a suggestion of a potential disease-free advantage in patients who had medially located primary tumors and axillary metastases, those patients most likely to have IM node involvement when these areas were subjected to treatment. Moreover, a large retrospective review from the British-Columbia Cancer Agency[25] found a poor overall survival and distant metastases-free survival in high-risk women who had medial tumors, again indicating the presence of untreated IM disease. Despite an overall trend to less extensive surgery, interest in the detection and treatment of IM nodes has resurfaced in recent years. The accurate evaluation and diagnosis of IM metastases is of importance in radiation treatment planning. Studies have consistently demonstrated that FDG-PET is better than CT in the detection of IM and mediastinal lymph nodal metastases (**Fig. 1**). In 73 consecutive patients who had recurrent or metastatic disease, PET was able to correctly identify 40% of the patients who had intrathoracic lymph node metastases, resulting in a sensitivity of 85% and a specificity of 90%.[26] Only 23% of the patients had suspiciously enlarged lymph nodes in CT, leading to a sensitivity of 54% and a specificity of 85%. Therefore, the overall diagnostic accuracy of PET (88%) was higher than that of CT (73%).[26] In patients with locally advanced breast cancer, the prevalence of IM FDG uptake can be as high as 25%.[27] The potential importance of IM nodal drainage has also been brought to the forefront with the widespread use of axillary sentinel node mapping, which frequently shows IM lymph drainage on lymphoscintigraphy. There is some speculation that a subset of patients who have "sternal metastases" may in fact be IM node failures with erosion of the sternum. If this is detected at initial diagnosis, the sternum can be effectively targeted with conformal radiation techniques. Although this approach can change the radiation field in some patients, the authors do not have outcome studies to suggest that this approach can improve the outcome.

The other area where PET/CT can potentially change the radiation field is the locally advanced breast cancer in which some studies have suggested a more posterior or medial location of lymph nodes than what is covered by a conventional supraclavicular field. In a study from MD Anderson Cancer Center, the investigators identified 33 patients with advanced or metastatic breast cancer who had a PET/CT scan demonstrating hypermetabolic supraclavicular lymph nodes.[28] The locations of the involved lymph nodes were mapped onto a single CT set of images of the supraclavicular fossa. These lymph nodes were also mapped onto the treatment-planning CT data set of 4 patients treated in the author's institution (2 patients with biopsy-proven supraclavicular nodes and 2 patients with clinically negative supraclavicular nodes). The results suggested that supraclavicular nodes can sometimes be posterior or medial to typical treatment volumes and could thus be underdosed. The drawback of the study was that most patients in this study had metastatic disease at the time of the PET/CT scan, and it is unclear whether these findings are applicable to patients with localized disease being treated to the supraclavicular field for presumed micrometastatic disease.

PET/CT can probably help in detection of disease in the supraclavicular region in some of these patients with locoregionally advanced breast cancer and can change the treatment

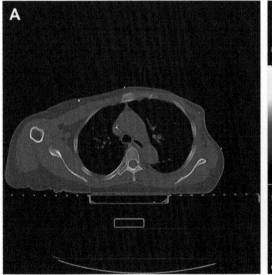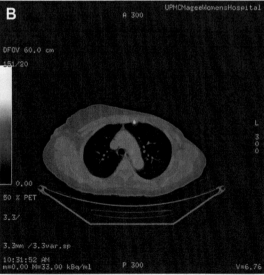

Fig. 1. (*A, B*) FDG-avid IM node seen on PET/CT while corresponding CT scan was read as normal.

volume and avoid geographic miss, thus potentially improving the outcome.

RADIATION THERAPY FOR ISOLATED LOCOREGIONAL RECURRENCE AFTER MASTECTOMY

FDG-PET can contribute in significant ways to the clinical management and radiation planning of patients who have suspected locoregional recurrences. The most common sites of locoregional recurrence among patients treated with mastectomy and axillary node dissection are chest wall and supraclavicular nodes. Because it provides biologic and functional information, FDG-PET is often complementary to conventional staging methods such as physical examination or cross-sectional imaging (CT or MR imaging), which rely more on changes in morphology to detect disease recurrence. These patients who have locoregional recurrences are at high risk for synchronous or metachronous distant metastases and need to be evaluated by a sensitive test that would change the management and outcome. Van Oost and colleagues[27] corroborated the need for a more sensitive staging tool in patients who have first-episode locoregional recurrence. In their study of 175 patients, they found that 16% had distant metastases at the time of locoregional recurrence and 24% developed distant metastases within 18 months of confirmation of recurrent disease. They estimated that FDG-PET would upstage and likely change the therapeutic plan in up to 29% of patients who have negative conventional staging studies. Besides, it can help to better define the extent of locoregional recurrence, which could change the radiation volume and dose.

PET can also be useful in evaluation of anatomic regions that have been previously treated by surgery or radiation, in which the discrimination between posttreatment scar and recurrent tumor is often problematic. Brachial plexopathy, for example, is difficult to assess on conventional anatomic imaging. FDG-PET and MR imaging were compared in 10 patients who had clinical findings suggestive of breast cancer metastases.[29] Out of 9 patients who had locoregional breast cancer metastases, MR imaging was positive in 5 patients and indeterminate in 4 patients, whereas FDG-PET was positive in all patients. Similar results were found in 19 patients with breast cancer who had symptoms referable to the brachial plexus, and it was concluded that FDG-PET may be particularly useful in distinguishing between radiation-induced and metastatic plexopathy.[30]

RADIATION THERAPY FOR METASTATIC DISEASE

The treatment techniques for palliative treatment usually treat a large volume for control of symptoms and have a limited role of PET/CT for planning in routine palliative radiation for breast cancer. There is an emerging role of radiation therapy for oligometastases. Oligometastatic disease represents a hypothesized state of metastatic progression in which a limited metastatic spread of disease is potentially curable with local therapy. The term "oligometastases," literally interpreted as "few metastases," was coined by Hellman and Weichselbaum in 1995.[31] Oligometastases has been hypothesized to represent a state of distant metastases in which local therapy, such as resection or radiation, may offer a cure in some patients.[31–35] Local control of oligometastatic lesions may also slow or prevent further metastatic progression.[36] Several institutions have been using hypofractionated stereotactic body radiotherapy (SBRT) or stereotactic radiosurgery (SRS) to treat oligometastases.[37–39]

Stereotactic radiotherapy uses a 3D coordinate system for accurate and reproducible patient setup and tumor localization. A system is needed to detect and process this 3D array. SBRT can be achieved through the use of internal fiducials, external markers, and/or image guidance. SBRT is advantageous in the treatment of oligometastatic disease, because aggressive fractionation can allow for improved disease control with acceptable toxicity. In a small prospective study evaluating SBRT for limited metastases from breast cancer treated with curative intent, the 4-year actuarial outcomes were overall survival of 59%, progression-free survival of 38%, and lesion local control of 89%.[40] On univariate analyses, 1 metastatic lesion (vs 2–5), smaller tumor volume, bone-only disease, and stable or regressing lesions before SBRT were associated with more favorable outcomes. SBRT has the potential to prolong survival and perhaps cure selected patients with limited metastases. The accurate targeting for SBRT or SRS becomes critical as higher dose per fraction is delivered, and better delineation of target can help improve local control and reduce the dose to critical organs. There are small studies in the literature suggesting that target delineation is better with integration of PET/CT for stereotactic radiation.[41,42] Large prospective studies are needed to evaluate the role of SBRT or SRS in oligometastases with integration of PET for staging and planning in patients with oligometastases. Prospective studies are needed to compare volumetric dose planning for target definition with radiosurgical treatment planning using FDG-PET and PET/CT, with currently used CT and MR imaging. For potential clinical application, it is important to demonstrate that the metabolic information is different from the anatomic tumor delineation and that it provides specific additional information. It also has to be shown that the ability to tailor radiation doses to a specific metabolic activity, as opposed to using conventional doses based on histology alone, results in improved local control. It is also important to determine specific features of FDG-PET and PET/CT that would predict local failure to standard radiosurgical dose prescriptions.

From the author's perspective, there is no doubt that FDG-PET/CT will become an important part of modern radiation treatment planning in the near future; however, it should be emphasized that currently FDG-PET can only be used as a complementary imaging modality for detecting disease that is not identified by CT.[43] The routine use of FDG-PET or PET/CT for radiation treatment planning requires a thorough and careful evaluation in large prospective studies as it relates to the promise of improving local control or increasing disease-free and overall survival.

PET/CT-based imaging is a valuable and useful test in the staging and restaging of breast cancer, especially in patients who have recurrent or locally advanced breast cancer. Its greatest clinical applications are in detection and definition of the extent of recurrent or metastatic disease. The role of PET/CT in radiation treatment planning for breast cancer is still in the nascent stages; controlled randomized trials data are lacking, and it is based on very few reported data. However, the potential to improve radiation treatment planning by allowing for the tailoring of comprehensive radiation portals, particularly for locally advanced or recurrent breast cancer, makes this one of the most promising tools in the era of image-guided radiation therapy.

CASE 1

A 47-year-old woman who had mastectomy done for stage IIA cancer noticed a nodule in her chest wall region. Biopsy result was consistent with recurrent disease. The PET/CT showed enlarged PET-avid interpectoral, deltoid region, and IM nodes, with no other site of metastatic disease (**Fig. 2**A). She was treated with chemotherapy with good response, followed by radiation to chest wall, IM, supraclavicular, and axillary region with modification of fields to cover all the aforementioned sites, followed by cone down boost to the site of initial gross disease to a total of 60 Gy (see **Fig. 2**B, C).

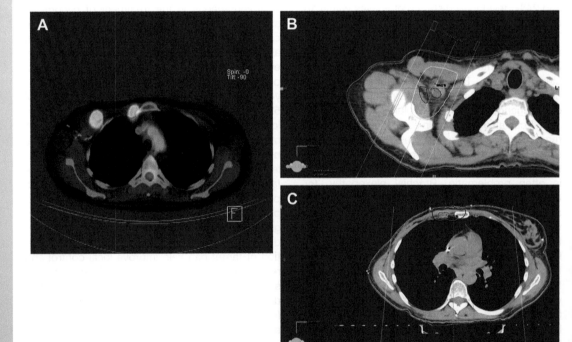

Fig. 2. (*A*) PET-CT showing recurrence in interpectoral node and IM node. (*B*) CT axial view showing single oblique beam covering recurrent node (*blue*) with prescription isodose line (*yellow*). (*C*) CT axial view showing single direct beam covering IM node (*red*) with prescription isodose line (*blue*).

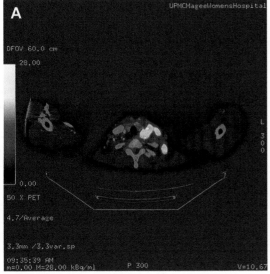

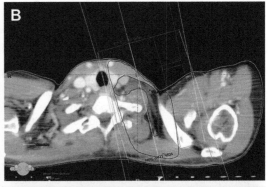

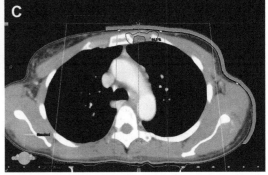

Fig. 3. (A) PET/CT showing enlarged FDG-avid nodes in supraclavicular region involving level V and medial level IV nodes. (B) CT axial view showing clinical target volume (red) covered by conformal anteroposterior-posteroanterior beam and prescription isodose line (blue). (C) CT axial view showing coverage of IM node (red) by single direct electron beam and prescription isodose line (blue).

CASE 2

A 52-year-old woman with locally advanced breast cancer with pretreatment PET/CT (Fig. 3A) with enlarged axillary, supraclavicular, and IM nodes treated, with neoadjuvant chemotherapy with good response, followed by modified radical mastectomy and axillary lymph node dissection. She then had radiation to chest wall, supraclavicular, and IM region. The supraclavicular nodes, as seen on PET/CT images, involve level V nodes posteriorly, which would not have been adequately covered with conventional fields, and the nodes needed field modification to cover them adequately (see Fig. 3B). Besides a separate field was also added to cover IM nodes (see Fig. 3C).

REFERENCES

1. Bucci MK, Bevan A, Roach M 3rd. Advances in radiation therapy: conventional to 3D, to IMRT, to 4D, and beyond. CA Cancer J Clin 2005;55(2):117–34.

2. Jansen EP, Dewit LG, van Herk M, et al. Target volumes in radiotherapy for high-grade malignant glioma of the brain. Radiother Oncol 2000;56(2): 151–6.

3. Quon A, Gambhir SS. FDG-PET and beyond: molecular breast cancer imaging. J Clin Oncol 2005;23(8): 1664–73.

4. American Cancer Society. Breast cancer facts & figures 2007–2008. Atlanta (GA): American Cancer Society; 2008.

5. Recht A, Edge SB, Solin LJ, et al. Postmastectomy radiotherapy: clinical practice guidelines of the American Society of Clinical Oncology. J Clin Oncol 2001;19(5):1539–69.

6. Jacobson JA, Danforth DN, Cowan KH, et al. Ten-year results of a comparison of conservation with mastectomy in the treatment of stage I and II breast cancer. N Engl J Med 1995;332(14):907–11.

7. van Dongen JA, Bartelink H, Fentiman IS, et al. Randomized clinical trial to assess the value of breast-conserving therapy in stage I and II breast cancer. EORTC 10801 trial. J Natl Cancer Inst Monogr 1992;11:15–8.

8. Sarrazin D, Le MG, Arriagada R, et al. Ten-year results of a randomized trial comparing a conservative treatment to mastectomy in early breast cancer. Radiother Oncol 1989;14(3):177–84.

9. Blichert-Toft M, Rose C, Anderson JA, et al. Danish randomized trial comparing breast conservation therapy with mastectomy. Six years of life-table analysis. J Natl Cancer Inst Monogr 1992;11:19–25.

10. Veronesi U, Banfi A, Salvadori B, et al. Breast conservation is the treatment of choice in small breast cancer. Long-term results of a randomized trial. Eur J Cancer 1990;26(6):668–70.

11. Fisher B, Anderson S, Redmond C, et al. Reanalysis and results after 12 years of followup in a randomized clinical trial comparing total mastectomy with lumpectomy with or without irradiation in the treatment of breast cancer. N Engl J Med 1995; 333(22):1456–61.

12. Cuzick J, Stewart H, Rutqvist L, et al. Cause specific mortality in long-term survivors of breast cancer who participated in trials of radiotherapy. J Clin Oncol 1994;12(3):447–53.

13. Gao X, Fisher S, Emami B. Risk of second primary cancer in the contralateral breast in women treated for early stage breast cancer: a population based study. Int J Radiat Oncol Biol Phys 2003;56: 1038–45.

14. Bhatnagar AK, Brandner E, Sonnik D, et al. Intensity-modulated radiation therapy (IMRT) reduces the dose to the contralateral breast when compared to conventional tangential fields for primary breast irradiation: initial report. Cancer J 2004;10(6):381–5.

15. Pierce LJ, Butler JB, Martel MK, et al. Postmastectomy radiotherapy of the chest wall: dosimetric comparison of common techniques. Int J Radiat Oncol Biol Phys 2002;52(5):1220–30.

16. Bradley J, Thorstad WL, Mutic S, et al. Impact of FDG-PET on radiation therapy volume delineation in non-small-cell lung cancer. Int J Radiat Oncol Biol Phys 2004;59(1):78–86.

17. Heron DE, Andrade RS, Flickinger J, et al. Hybrid PET-CT simulation for radiation treatment planning in head-and-neck cancers: a brief technical report. Int J Radiat Oncol Biol Phys 2004;60(5):1419–24.

18. Ford EC, Lavely WC, Frassica DA, et al. Comparison of FDG-PET/CT and CT for delineation of lumpectomy cavity for partial breast irradiation. Int J Radiat Oncol Biol Phys 2008;71(2):595–602.

19. Overgaard M, Hansen PS, Overgaard J, et al. Post-operative radiotherapy in high-risk premenopausal women with breast cancer who receive adjuvant chemotherapy. Danish Breast Cancer Cooperative Group 82b Trial. N Engl J Med 1997;337(14): 949–55.

20. Ragaz J, Jackson SM, Le N, et al. Adjuvant radiotherapy and chemotherapy in node-positive premenopausal women with breast cancer. N Engl J Med 1997;337(14):956–62.

21. Overgaard M, Jensen MB, Overgaard J, et al. Postoperative radiotherapy in high-risk postmenopausal breast-cancer patients given adjuvant tamoxifen: Danish Breast Cancer Cooperative Group DBCG 82c randomised trial. Lancet 1999;353(9165):1641–8.

22. Lacour J, Le M, Caceres E, et al. Radical mastectomy versus radical mastectomy plus internal mammary dissection. Ten year results of an international cooperative trial in breast cancer. Cancer 1983;51:1941–3.

23. Veronesi U, Valagussa P. Inefficacy of internal mammary node dissection in breast cancer surgery. Cancer 1981;47:170–5.

24. Lacour J, Le MG, Hill C. Is it useful to remove internal mammary nodes in operable breast cancer? Eur J Surg Oncol 1987;13:309–14.

25. Lohrisch C, Jackson J, Jones A, et al. Relationship between tumor location and relapse in 6781 women with early invasive breast cancer. J Clin Oncol 2000; 18:2828–35.

26. Eubank WB, Mankoff DA, Takasugi J. 18Fluoro-deoxyglucose positron emission tomography to detect mediastinal or internal mammary metastases in breast cancer. J Clin Oncol 2001;19: 3516–23.

27. van Oost FJ, van der Hoeven JJ, Hoekstra OS. Staging in patients with locoregionally recurrent breast cancer: current practice and prospects for positron emission tomography. Eur J Cancer 2004; 40:1545–53.

28. Reed VK, Cavalcanti JL, Strom EA, et al. Risk of subclinical micrometastatic disease in the supraclavicular nodal bed according to the anatomic distribution in patients with advanced breast cancer. Int J Radiat Oncol Biol Phys 2008;71(2): 435–40.

29. Hathaway PB, Mankoff DA, Maravilla KR, et al. Value of combined FDG PET and MR imaging in the evaluation of suspected recurrent localregional breast cancer: preliminary experience. Radiology 1999; 210(3):807–14.

30. Ahmad A, Barrington S, Maisey M, et al. Use of positron emission tomography in evaluation of brachial plexopathy in breast cancer patients. Br J Cancer 1999;79(3–4):478–82.

31. Hellman S, Weichselbaum RR. Oligometastases. J Clin Oncol 1995;13:8–10.

32. Milano MT, Katz AW, Muhs AG, et al. A prospective pilot study of curative-intent stereotactic body radiation therapy in patients with 5 or fewer oligometastatic lesions. Cancer 2008;112:650–8.

33. Hellman S, Weichselbaum RR. Importance of local control in an era of systemic therapy. Nat Clin Pract Oncol 2005;2:60–1.

34. Koong AC, Le QT, Ho A, et al. Phase I study of stereotactic radiosurgery in patients with locally advanced pancreatic cancer. Int J Radiat Oncol Biol Phys 2004;58:1017–21.

35. Tait CR, Waterworth A, Loncaster J, et al. The oligometastatic state in breast cancer: hypothesis or reality. Breast 2005;14:87–93.

36. Withers HR, Lee SP. Modeling growth kinetics and statistical distribution of oligometastases. Semin Radiat Oncol 2006;16:111–9.

37. Sampson MC, Katz A, Constine LS. Stereotactic body radiation therapy for extracranial oligometastases: does the sword have a double edge? Semin Radiat Oncol 2006;16:67–76.

38. Kavanagh BD, McGarry RC, Timmerman RD. Extracranial radiosurgery (stereotactic body radiation therapy) for oligometastases. Semin Radiat Oncol 2006;16:77–84.

39. Timmerman RD, Kavanagh BD, Cho LC, et al. Stereotactic body radiation therapy in multiple organ sites. J Clin Oncol 2007;25:947–52.

40. Milano MT, Katz AW, Schell MC, et al. Descriptive analysis of oligometastatic lesions treated with curative-intent stereotactic body radiotherapy. Int J Radiat Oncol Biol Phys 2008;72(5):1516–22.

41. Gwak HS, Youn SM, Chang U, et al. Usefulness of (18)F-fluorodeoxyglucose PET for radiosurgery planning and response monitoring in patients with recurrent spinal metastasis. Minim Invasive Neurosurg 2006;49(3):127–34.

42. Coon D, Gokhale AS, Burton SA, et al. Fractionated stereotactic body radiation therapy in the treatment of primary, recurrent, and metastatic lung tumors: the role of positron emission tomography/computed tomography-based treatment planning. Clin Lung Cancer 2008;9(4):217–21.

43. Heron DE, Andrade RS, Beriwal S, et al. PET-CT in radiation oncology: the impact on diagnosis, treatment planning, and assessment of treatment response. Am J Clin Oncol 2008;31(4):352–62.

PET and PET-CT Imaging in Treatment Monitoring of Breast Cancer

Rakesh Kumar, MD[a],*, Madhavi Chawla, MD[a],
Sandip Basu, MBBS (Hons), DRM, DNB, MNAMS[b],
Abass Alavi, MD, MD (Hon), PhD (Hon), DSc (Hon)[c]

KEYWORDS
• Breast cancer • ^{18}F-FDG PET • Tumor • Chemotherapy

Breast cancer is the most frequently diagnosed cancer in women. It remains the second most frequent cause of cancer death after lung and bronchial cancers in women worldwide. Breast cancer is one of the more responsive solid tumors,[1] for which a wide range of systemic therapy options are available. Therefore, appropriate evaluation of early response to therapy is an important diagnostic need for breast cancer. The treatment of newly diagnosed breast cancer is primarily determined by the extent of disease and generally includes surgery, radiation, and chemotherapy. Primary systemic chemotherapy or neoadjuvant chemotherapy, introduced for managing inoperable and large or locally advanced breast tumors,[2] is now increasingly being used to downstage tumor load before surgery. This renders previously inoperable breast cancer resectable, permitting breast-conserving surgery and sentinel node biopsy instead of subsequent axillary lymph node dissection.[3–5] The therapeutic options available for patients with metastatic breast cancer are various,[6,7] depending on the histopathology and the extent of disease. Patients with estrogen receptor–positive tumors and a small volume of metastatic disease are treated with endocrine agents,[7] patients with HER2-positive tumors are treated with a combination of trastuzumab and chemotherapy,[8] and the only current treatment option available for patients with triple-negative tumors (ie, estrogen-negative, progesterone-negative, and HER2-negative tumors) is chemotherapy.[9]

IMAGING MODALITIES EVALUATING TREATMENT RESPONSE IN BREAST CANCER

Various imaging modalities are available for staging, restaging and response evaluation in oncology. Standard imaging techniques for breast carcinoma include radiologic examinations, such as x-ray mammography, Doppler ultrasonography,[10] computed tomography (CT), magnetic resonance imaging (MRI), magnetic resonance spectroscopy,[11,12] and optical imaging.[13] Among these functional imaging modalities, contrast-enhanced MRI is the most widely used in clinical practice, as it provides a detailed anatomic picture of the extent of disease, which is important for surgical planning after therapy.[14] Combining MRI and contrast-enhanced MRI has a diagnostic accuracy of 93% for identifying tumors showing a pathologic complete response (pCR).[15] Nuclear medicine techniques also play an important role in diagnosing and staging breast cancer. In the past, only bone scintigraphy was used to detect bone metastases at an early stage.[16] This technique was followed by imaging using monoclonal

[a] Department of Nuclear Medicine, All India Institute of Medical Sciences, New Delhi 110029, India
[b] Radiation Medicine Centre, Bhabha Atomic Research Centre, Mumbai, India
[c] Nuclear Medicine Section, Radiology Department, Hospital of the University of Pennsylvania, Philadelphia, PA, USA
* Corresponding author.
E-mail address: rkphulia@hotmail.com (R. Kumar).

PET Clin 4 (2009) 359–369
doi:10.1016/j.cpet.2009.09.008
1556-8598/09/$ – see front matter © 2009 Elsevier Inc. All rights reserved.

antibodies against carcinoembryonic antigens and other antigens expressed in breast cancer and imaging with ^{99m}Tc-tetrofosmin or ^{99m}Tc-sestamibi for primary and recurrent disease.[17,18] Since the introduction of positron emission tomography (PET) in clinical oncology, ^{18}F-fluorodeoxyglucose (^{18}F-FDG) PET has been shown to be an effective and accurate imaging modality for staging and re-staging of recurrent and metastatic disease and for treatment monitoring.[19–22]

Treatment Response Evaluation of Primary Breast Cancer

Sequential ^{18}F-FDG PET imaging has been widely studied as a method for assessing tumor response to neoadjuvant chemotherapy. The concept of using ^{18}F-FDG PET for predicting a therapeutic response is based on early changes in tumor glucose use and the close correlation of changes in ^{18}F-FDG uptake with the effectiveness of therapy.[23,24] In all these studies, ^{18}F-FDG PET scans were obtained before therapy and then at variable intervals during the course of neoadjuvant therapy (**Fig. 1**). Comparison of the levels of radiotracer uptake in the baseline scan and in subsequent posttherapy scans helped in early identification of responders and in differentiating them from the nonresponders. Currently there is

no definite consensus about the optimal timing of FDG PET, and studies have been performed at various points after chemotherapy. In most of these studies, a single scan was performed early during the course of treatment.[25–34] Other studies included 2 or 3 scans performed sequentially during the course of treatment.[23,35–42] Studies of FDG PET after the first cycle of chemotherapy have shown sensitivities ranging from 39% to 100%.[23,37,38,40] Specificities ranged from 74% to100%.[23,37,38,40] Corresponding range of sensitivities and specificities after the second cycle were 69% to93%[32,38,40] and 75% to94%,[32,38,40] respectively. Literature suggests that response evaluation is most effective after the second cycle (**Fig. 2**).[40] Evaluation of treatment response after the first cycle of chemotherapy will have lower accuracy, and evaluation after 3 or more cycles will be too late to make an effective alteration and the patient will already have been exposed to ineffective and toxic chemotherapy (**Table 1**).

ANALYSIS AND ASSESSMENT OF TUMOR RESPONSE TO THERAPY

Several methods for quantitative analysis of FDG data have been proposed.[44] In the dynamic scanning protocol, an attempt to measure glucose

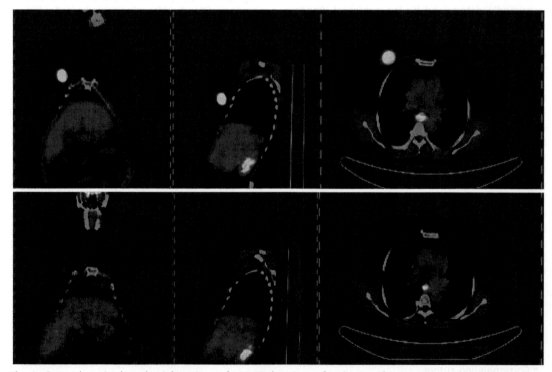

Fig. 1. Coronal, sagittal, and axial sections of PET-CT showing a focal area of intense increased FDG uptake in right breast in baseline PET-CT study (*top*). Follow-up study, after completion of chemotherapy, shows complete resolution of right breast tumor (*bottom*).

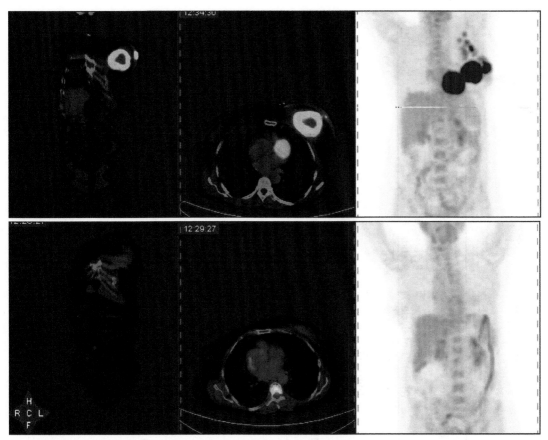

Fig. 2. Coronal, sagittal, and projection image of PET-CT showing a focal area of intense increased FDG uptake with central necrosis in left breast and multiple left axillary lymph nodes in baseline PET-CT study (*top*). Follow-up study, after completion of chemotherapy, shows complete resolution of right breast tumor and axillary lymph nodes (*bottom*).

metabolic rate is made. This protocol is, however, considered to be too time-consuming and technically demanding for routine clinical use, which has resulted in the development of methods that require just a single static scan. At present, the standard uptake value (SUV) method is most widely used. This method requires a single scan to measure the uptake of FDG, which is then normalized to injected dose and body weight. Normalization to body surface area or lean body mass can also be done.[45–48] Definition of the tumor region of interest for the calculation of SUV is of crucial importance in monitoring tumor uptake of FDG during therapy. Reproducibility, user independence, and, to a lesser degree, simplicity are important considerations when choosing a region-of-interest method.

In most studies, histopathologic assessment of response to therapy from the postsurgical specimen was used as the gold standard,[23,25,26,32,36–38,40–43] pCR being defined by the absence of residual invasive tumor.[49–51]

However, no difference was found in survival rates between patients with scattered microscopic foci of residual tumor cells and patients who achieved a pCR.[52] Thus both groups were classified together as minimal residual disease, all other responses being classified as gross residual disease. Other studies used clinical evaluation,[28,35] assessment of size by conventional imaging methods,[34,35] tumor marker levels,[27] recurrence rate, and mortality rate[31] as reference parameters.

Two important criteria, namely, the World Health Organization criteria[53] and RECIST (response evaluation criteria in solid tumors) criteria,[54] based on conventional imaging modalities, have been described in the literature to define the tumor response. Assessment of tumor size using RECIST criteria was the commonest among these. The RECIST criteria define a response as a decrease in the maximum tumor diameter of at least 30%.[54] Despite the wide acceptance of the above-mentioned criteria in clinical practice, there were a few limitations in evaluation of treatment

Table 1
Studies evaluating treatment response using PET/PET-CT in patients with breast cancer

Authors	Year	Number of Patients	Stage	Isotope	Serial PET (Number of Cycles)	Reference Standard	Sensitivity	Specificity
Wahl et al[23]	1993	11	IIIB/LABC	FDG	First (11) Second (11) Third (11)	HPR	100	100
Bruce et al[25]	1995	12	LABC	FDG	Second (5)	HPR	—	—
Janson et al[35]	1995	16	LABC/IV	FDG/ 11C MET	First (7) Third/fourth (7)	Clinical/ conventional Imaging	—	—
Bassa et al[36]	1996	16	LABC	FDG	Mid (13) Presurgery (14)	HPR	75	—
Smith et al[37]	2000	30	T3/LABC	FDG	First (28) Fourth (19) Eighth (21)	HPR	90	74
Schelling et al[38]	2000	22	LABC	FDG	First (14) Second (20)	HPR	100 83	85 94
Tiling et al[39]	2001	7	LABC	FDG	Day 8 (7) Second (7)		—	—
Mankoff et al[26]	2003	35	LABC	FDG/ ^{15}O-H_2O	Mid (21)	Tumor size HPR	—	—
Kim et al[43]	2004	50	LABC		Complete (50)	HPR	85	83
Rousseau et al[40]	2006	64	II/III	FDG	First (64) Second (64) Third (64)	HPR	39 69 79	96 89 77
Pio et al[27]	2006	14	Primary/ metastatic	FLT	First (14)	CA27.29 CT	—	—
Kenny et al[28]	2007	13	II–IV	FLT	First (13)	Clinical response	—	—
McDermott et al[41]	2007	NA	LABC	FDG	First Mid	HPR	100	77

Li D et al[29]	2007	45		FDG	Third (45)	MR spectroscopy	91	83
Tozakiet et al[30]	2008	7		FDG	Mid		
Dunnwald et al[31]	2008	53	LABC	FDG/^{15}O-H$_2$O	Mid	Recurrence Mortality rate	
Kumar et al[32]	2009	23	LABC	FDG	Second	HPR	93
Schwarz-Dose[42]	2009	104	LABC	FDG	First (87) Second (81)	HPR	75

Abbreviations: FLT, fluorothymidine; HPR, histopathology response; LABC, locally advanced breast cancer; MET, methionine; NA, not available.

response. An important limitation is the assumption that the chemotherapy agent under review is cytocidal and that it will lead to cell death followed by reduction in tumor size. The cut off criteria of 50% or 30% reduction in tumor size are arbitrary percentages and are not based on outcome studies. Several cycles of treatment are needed before a change in tumor size can be assessed by anatomic imaging. This approach works well for some sites of metastatic disease, such as the liver and lungs, but regional nodal disease and bones are difficult to evaluate.[55] These limitations of CT/MRI can be effectively overcome by functional imaging techniques, which have the unique ability to detect subclinical alterations in tumor physiology and biochemistry resulting from efficacious therapy.[56] Besides this, ^{18}F-FDG PET also identified patients with low tumor metabolic activity before treatment as not achieving histopathologic response, suggesting that breast cancers with low metabolic activity are not likely to respond to primary chemotherapy, thus guiding initial management.[40–42,57]

TREATMENT RESPONSE EVALUATION IN METASTATIC DISEASE

The presence of residual tumor in axillary lymph nodes after chemotherapy is an independent risk factor for locoregional recurrence in locally advanced breast cancer (LABC).[58,59] However, response monitoring data on the axillary status are scarce. Only 3 studies have looked specifically at response of axillary lymph nodes. Smith and colleagues[37] found a significantly greater mean decrease in FDG uptake after 1 cycle of therapy in lymph nodes with pathologic microscopic residual disease than in nonresponding nodes. Bassa and colleagues[36] and Buscombe and colleagues[60] reported sensitivities for detecting residual lymph node involvement after completion of therapy of 42% and 40%, respectively. Specificity was 100% in both studies. Studies performed after the completion of chemotherapy have shown that although residual ^{18}F-FDG uptake predicts residual disease, the absence of ^{18}F-FDG uptake is not a reliable indicator of pCR.[36,60–62] This is especially true for axillary nodal disease, because the sensitivity for residual microscopic disease after therapy is low. There is a relative paucity of studies that had evaluated the role of metastatic disease other than bone and axillary lymph nodes (**Fig. 3**).

The bone is the most common site of distant metastasis, and metastases to the bone are diagnosed in 30% to 85% of patients with

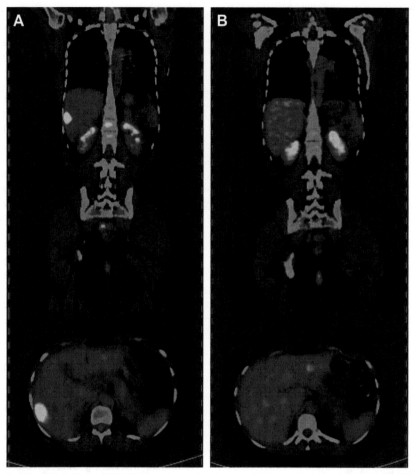

Fig. 3. Coronal and axial section of PET-CT showing a focal area of intense increased FDG uptake in liver suggestive of metastasis in a patient with breast cancer (*A*). Follow-up study, after 6 cycles of chemotherapy, shows resolution of liver lesion (*B*).

advanced breast cancer.[63] Bone metastasis causes much of the morbidity and disability in patients with breast cancer because of its potentially prolonged clinical course. Relatively small studies have been conducted evaluating serial ^{18}F-FDG PET for measuring metastatic breast cancer response to treatment. Most studies concluded that response is accompanied by substantial drops in ^{18}F-FDG uptake, typically 40% to 50% or more from the pretherapy baseline scans.[64–66] Most studies evaluated response after the first cycle of chemotherapy.[27,28,33,66] Additional scans were performed after the second,[65] third,[64] or third/fourth[35] cycle in some studies. Clinical response,[28,35,64] conventional imaging,[27,35,65] tumor markers,[27] circulating tumor cell counts, and survival rates[67] were used as the reference standards in patients with bone metastasis. Some studies suggested that imaging as early as after 1 cycle of chemotherapy could predict response,[66] akin to the neoadjuvant therapy setting. However, other studies have not shown similar accuracy for early repeated ^{18}F-FDG PET.[64] Even though favorable results have been reported, prospective, multicenter clinical trials are needed to validate the efficacy for ^{18}F-FDG PET/CT for evaluating bone metastasis response and to enable their more widespread clinical use in bone-dominant breast cancer (**Table 2**).

FLARE PHENOMENON IN THE SCENARIO OF THERAPEUTIC RESPONSE IN BREAST CARCINOMA

Although FDG PET has been a highly successful modality in monitoring response to treatment, tumor recurrence, and restaging, one must keep in mind the phenomenon of "metabolic flare,"

Table 2
Studies evaluating treatment response using PET/PET-CT in patients with metastatic breast cancer

Authors	Year	Number of Patients	Isotope	Serial PET (Number of Cycles)	Reference Standard
Jansson et al[35]	1995	4	FDG/ ^{11}C-MET	First Third/fourth	Clinical/conventional imaging
Gennari et al[66]	2000	9	FDG	First	
Dose Schwarz et al[65]	2005	11	FDG	First Second	Conventional imaging
Pio et al[27]	2006	14	FLT	First (14)	CA27.29 CT
Couturier et al[64]	2006	20	FDG	First Third	Clinical response
Specht et al[78]	2007	28	FDG	Mid	
Kenny et al[28]	2007	13	FLT	First (13)	Clinical response
Lindholm et al[33]	2009	13	^{11}C-MET	First	
DeGiorgi et al[67]	2009	115	FDG	Mid	Circulating tumor cell count Patient survival

Abbreviations: FLT, fluorothymidine; MET, methionine.

which is a transient increase in FDG activity very early in the course of therapy. Such an increase occurs 7 to 10 days after initiating hormonal therapy because of partial estrogen-like agonist effects of tamoxifen and should not be construed as disease progression. Metabolic flare also occurs after radiation/systemic therapy because of the accumulation of inflammatory cells at the treatment site.

TREATMENT RESPONSE EVALUATION WITH OTHER TRACERS

Studies of ^{18}F-FDG PET have shown that tumor glycolysis declines early in the course of treatment,[37,38] providing a means for early response assessment. However, other pathways more closely related to perfusion, cellular growth, and death may provide even earlier and more specific indications of therapeutic response. Tumor perfusion may influence response to systemic chemotherapy[68] and good perfusion is crucial for the delivery of chemotherapy to the tumor cell,[69] which is evaluated using ^{15}O-water PET.[70] Tumors with low perfusion may be hypoxic, and hypoxia has been related to aggressive tumor behavior and poor response to chemotherapy.[71] Mankoff and colleagues[26] and Dunnwald and colleagues[31] used ^{15}O-water for midcycle assessment of response to therapy in patients with LABC and have shown that serial measures of breast cancer perfusion by ^{15}O-water PET in the neoadjuvant setting are highly predictive of response and survival. Some studies have suggested that dynamic ^{18}F-FDG PET and

kinetic analysis may yield estimates of tumor perfusion, inferred from the ^{18}F-FDG delivery kinetic parameter, comparable to ^{15}O-water PET.[72–74] This approach, therefore, merits further investigation. **Table 3** lists the studies done with PET radiopharmaceuticals other than FDG.

The uptake of labeled amino acids, such as ^{11}C-methionine (MET), correlates with tumor growth, and changes in uptake provide an early indication of breast cancer response to therapy. Jansson and colleagues[35] performed ^{11}C-MET PET in 11 patients with LABC/stage IV, either alone or in conjunction with FDG PET, after the first and the third/fourth course of chemotherapy. Clinical evaluation and conventional imaging were used as the reference standards. A similar study after the first cycle was performed by Lindholm and colleagues[33] in 13 patients with metastatic breast carcinoma. Both the studies showed changes in uptake, providing an early indication of breast cancer response to therapy.[35]

Aberrant cellular proliferation can be studied using ^{18}F-fluorothymidine (^{18}F-FLT). Response evaluation after a single cycle of chemotherapy in patients with primary/metastatic disease has been studied by Pio and colleagues[27] and Kenny and colleagues[28] in 14 and 13 patients, respectively, and appears especially promising for measuring the early effects of therapy on breast cancer growth.

16α-^{18}F-fluoro-17β-estradiol (^{18}F-FES)[75] PET appears to be a promising tracer for noninvasively determining the estrogen receptor status of metastatic breast cancer and predicting the response

Table 3
Studies evaluating treatment response using isotopes other than FDG in patients with primary/metastatic breast cancer

Authors	Year	Number of Patients	Stage	Isotope	Serial PET (Number of Cycles)	Reference Standard
Jansson et al[35]	1995	16	LABC/IV	FDG/ ^{11}C-MET	First (7) Third (7)	Conventional imaging
Mankoff et al[26]	2003	35	LABC	FDG/ ^{15}O-H_2O	Mid (21)	Tumor size HPR
Pio et al[27]	2006	14	Primary/ metastatic	FLT	First (14)	CA27.29 CT
Kenny et al[28]	2007	13	II-IV	FLT	First (13)	Clinical response
Dunnwald et al[31]	2008	53	LABC	FDG/ ^{15}O-H_2O	Mid	Recurrence Mortality rate
Lindholm et al[33]	2009	13	Metastatic	^{11}C-MET	First	

Abbreviations: FLT, fluorothymidine; HPR, histopathology response; MET, methionine.

to endocrine therapy. Similarly, HER2 (ErbB2) expression in breast cancer is an important indicator of prognosis and an increasingly important target for therapy.[76] Studies using a ^{68}Ga-labeled F(ab9)2 fragment of trastuzumab[77] demonstrated the feasibility of measuring regional HER2 expression in murine animal models. However, further studies are merited before these radiotracers are put into clinical use.

SUMMARY

Breast cancer is a more responsive solid tumor with a wide range of systemic therapy options. The early identification of nonresponders is important because the availability of newer chemotherapy agents helps in avoiding expensive, ineffective, and toxic drugs and because of the possibility to switch over to alternative treatment methods. ^{18}F-FDG, being a glucose analog, can predict therapeutic response based on early changes in tumor glucose use, which correlates well with the effectiveness of treatment. ^{18}F-FDG PET thus serves as an effective and accurate imaging modality for staging and restaging of recurrent and metastatic disease, and early treatment monitoring.

ACKNOWLEDGMENTS

This work also was supported in part by the Council of Scientific and Industrial Research, New Delhi, India under Senior Research Associate Fellowship.

REFERENCES

1. Gralow JR. Optimizing the treatment of metastatic breast cancer. Breast Cancer Res Treat 2005; 89(Suppl 1):S9–15.
2. Bonadonna G, Valagussa P, Zucali R, et al. Primary chemotherapy in surgically resectable breast cancer. CA Cancer J Clin 1995;45:227–43.
3. Moneer M, Ismael S, Khaled H, et al. A new surgical strategy for breast conservation in locally advanced breast cancer that achieves a good locoregional control rate: preliminary report. Breast 2001;10: 220–4.
4. Stearns V, Ewing CA, Slack R, et al. Sentinel lymphadenectomy after neoadjuvant chemotherapy for breast cancer may reliably represent the axilla except for inflammatory breast cancer. Ann Surg Oncol 2002;9:235–42.
5. Breslin TM, Cohen L, Sahin A, et al. Sentinel lymph node biopsy is accurate after neoadjuvant chemotherapy for breast cancer. J Clin Oncol 2000;18: 3480–6.
6. Hamilton A, Hortobagyi G. Chemotherapy: what progress in the last 5 years? J Clin Oncol 2005;23: 1760–75.
7. Higgins MJ, Wolff AC. Therapeutic options in the management of metastatic breast cancer. Oncology 2008;22:614–23.
8. Ligibel JA, Winer EP. Trastuzumab/chemotherapy combinations in metastatic breast cancer. Semin Oncol 2002;29:38–43.
9. Kilburn LS. 'Triple negative' breast cancer: a new area for phase III breast cancer clinical trials. Clin Oncol 2008;20:35–9.
10. Kedar RP, Cosgrove DO, Smith IE, et al. Breast carcinoma: measurement of tumor response to

primary medical therapy with color flow Doppler imaging. Radiology 1994;190:825–30.

11. Bolan PJ, Nelson MT, Yee D, et al. Imaging in breast cancer: magnetic resonance spectroscopy. Breast Cancer Res 2005;7:149–52.

12. Lehman CD, Schnall MD. Imaging in breast cancer: magnetic resonance imaging. Breast Cancer Res 2005;7:215–9.

13. Tromberg BJ, Cerussi A, Shah N, et al. Imaging in breast cancer: diffuse optics in breast cancer—detecting tumors in pre-menopausal women and monitoring neoadjuvant chemotherapy. Breast Cancer Res 2005;7:279–85.

14. Hylton N. MR imaging for assessment of breast cancer response to neoadjuvant chemotherapy. Magn Reson Imaging Clin N Am 2006;14:383–9.

15. Martincich L, Montemurro F, De Rosa G, et al. Monitoring response to primary chemotherapy in breast cancer using dynamic contrast-enhanced magnetic resonance imaging. Breast Cancer Res Treat 2004; 83:67–76.

16. Cook G, Fogelman I. Skeletal metastases from breast cancer: imaging with nuclear medicine. Semin Nucl Med 1999;29:69–79.

17. Lind P, Gallowitsch H, Kogler D, et al. Tc-99m tetrofosmin mammoscintigraphy: a prospective study in primary breast lesions. Nucl Med 1996;35:225–9.

18. Spanu A, Farris A, Schillaci O, et al. The usefulness of Tc-99m tetrofosmin scintigraphy in patients with breast cancer recurrences. Nucl Med Commun 2003;24:145–54.

19. Flanagan F, Dehdashti F, Siegel B. PET in breast cancer. Semin Nucl Med 1998;28:290–302.

20. Avril N, Schelling M, Dose J, et al. Utility of PET in breast cancer. Clin Positron Imaging 1999;2:261–71.

21. Bombardieri E, Grippa F. PET imaging in breast cancer. Q J Nucl Med 2001;43:245–56.

22. Czernin J. FDG PET in breast cancer: a different view of its clinical use. Mol Imaging Biol 2002;4: 35–45.

23. Wahl RL, Zasadny K, Helvie M, et al. Metabolic monitoring of breast cancer chemohormonotherapy using positron emission tomography: initial evaluation. J Clin Oncol 1993;11:2101–11.

24. Weber WA. Positron emission tomography as an imaging biomarker. J Clin Oncol 2006;24: 3282–92.

25. Bruce DM, Evans NT, Heys SD, et al. Positron emission tomography: 2-deoxy-2 [18F]-fluoro-D-glucose uptake in locally advanced breast cancers. Eur J Surg Oncol 1995;21:280–3.

26. Mankoff DA, Dunnwald LK, Gralow JR, et al. Changes in blood flow and metabolism in locally advanced breast cancer treated with neoadjuvant chemotherapy. J Nucl Med 2003;44:1806–14.

27. Pio BS, Park CK, Pietras R, et al. Usefulness of 3'-[F-18] fluoro-3'-deoxythymidine with positron emission tomography in predicting breast cancer response to therapy. Mol Imaging Biol 2006;8:36–42.

28. Kenny L, Coombes RC, Vigushin DM, et al. Imaging early changes in proliferation at 1 week post chemotherapy: a pilot study in breast cancer patients with 3'-deoxy-3'-[18F] fluorothymidine positron emission tomography. Eur J Nucl Med Mol Imaging 2007; 34(9):1339–47.

29. Li D, Yao Q, Li L, et al. Correlation between hybrid 18F-FDG PET/CT and apoptosis induced by neoadjuvant chemotherapy in breast cancer. Cancer Biol Ther 2007;6:1442–8.

30. Tozaki M, Sakamoto M, Oyama Y, et al. Monitoring of early response to chemotherapy in breast cancer with (1)H MR spectroscopy: comparison to sequential 2-[18F]- fluorodeoxyglucose positron emission tomography. J Magn Reson Imaging 2008;28(2): 420–7.

31. Dunnwald LK, Gralow JR, Ellis GK, et al. Tumor metabolism and blood flow changes by positron emission tomography: relation to survival in patients treated with neoadjuvant chemotherapy for locally advanced breast cancer. J Clin Oncol 2008;26: 4449–57.

32. Kumar A, Kumar R, Seenu V, et al. The role of 18F FDG PET/CT in evaluation of early response to neoadjuvant chemotherapy in patients with locally advanced breast cancer. Eur Radiol 2009;19(6): 1347–57.

33. Lindholm P, Lapela M, Nagren K, et al. Preliminary study of carbon-11 methionine PET in the evaluation of early response to therapy in advanced breast cancer. Nucl Med Commun 2009;30(1):30–6.

34. Duch J, Fuster D, Munoz M, et al. 18F-FDG PET/CT for early prediction of response to neoadjuvant chemotherapy in breast cancer. Eur J Nucl Med. Mol Imaging 2009;36:1551–7.

35. Jansson T, Westlin JE, Ahlstrom H, et al. Positron emission tomography studies in patients with locally advanced and/or metastatic breast cancer: a method for early therapy evaluation? J Clin Oncol 1995;13:1470–7.

36. Bassa P, Kim E, Inoue T, et al. Evaluation of preoperative chemotherapy using PET with fluorine-18-fluorodeoxyglucose in breast cancer. J Nucl Med 1996;37:931–8.

37. Smith IC, Welch AE, Hutcheon AW, et al. Positron emission tomography using (18F)-fluorodeoxy-D-glucose to predict the pathologic response of breast cancer to primary chemotherapy. J Clin Oncol 2000; 18:1676–88.

38. Schelling M, Avril N, Nahrig J, et al. Positron emission tomography using [18F]fluorodeoxyglucose for monitoring primary chemotherapy in breast cancer. J Clin Oncol 2000;18:1689–95.

39. Tiling R, Linke R, Untch M, et al. 18F-FDG PET and 99mTc-sestamibi scintimammography for

monitoring breast cancer response to neoadjuvant chemotherapy: a comparative study. Eur J Nucl Med 2001;28:711–20.

40. Rousseau C, Devillers A, Sagan C, et al. Monitoring of early response to neoadjuvant chemotherapy in stage II and III breast cancer by [18F] fluorodeoxyglucose positron emission tomography. J Clin Oncol 2006;24: 5366–72.

41. McDermott GM, Welch A, Staff RT, et al. Monitoring primary breast cancer throughout chemotherapy using FDG-PET. Breast Cancer Res Treat 2007; 102(1):75–84.

42. Schwarz-Dose J, Untch M, Tiling R, et al. Monitoring primary systemic therapy of large and locally advanced breast cancer by using sequential positron emission tomography imaging with [18F]fluoro-deoxyglucose. J Clin Oncol 2009;27:535–41.

43. Kim SJ, Kim SK, Lee ES, et al. Predictive value of [18F] FDG PET for pathological response of breast cancer to neo-adjuvant chemotherapy. Ann Oncol 2004;15:1352–7.

44. Hoekstra CJ, Paglianiti I, Hoekstra OS, et al. Monitoring response to therapy in cancer using [18F]-2-fluoro-2-deoxy-Dglucose and positron emission tomography: an overview of different analytical methods. Eur J Nucl Med 2000;27:731–43.

45. Kim CK, Gupta NC, Chandramouli B, et al. Standardized uptake values of FDG: body surface area correction is preferable to body weight correction. J Nucl Med 1994;35:164–7.

46. Schomburg A, Bender H, Reichel C, et al. Standardized uptake values of fluorine-18 fluorodeoxyglucose: the value of different normalization procedures. Eur J Nucl Med 1996;23:571–4.

47. Sugawara Y, Zasadny KR, Neuhoff AW, et al. Reevaluation of the standardized uptake value for FDG: variations with body weight and methods for correction. Radiology 1999;213:521–5.

48. Erselcan T, Turgut B, Dogan D, et al. Lean body mass-based standardized uptake value, derived from a predictive equation, might be misleading in PET studies. Eur J Nucl Med Mol Imaging 2002;29:1630–8.

49. van der Hage JA, van de Velde CJ, Julien JP, et al. Preoperative chemotherapy in primary operable breast cancer: results from the European Organization for Research and Treatment of Cancer trial 10902. J Clin Oncol 2001;19:4224–37.

50. Bonadonna G, Valagussa P, Brambilla C, et al. Primary chemotherapy in operable breast cancer: eight-year experience at the Milan Cancer Institute. J Clin Oncol 1998;16:93–100.

51. Fisher ER, Wang J, Bryant J, et al. Pathobiology of preoperative chemotherapy: findings from the National Surgical Adjuvant Breast and Bowel (NSABP) protocol B-18. Cancer 2002;95:681–95.

52. Honkoop AH, van Diest PJ, de Jong JS, et al. Prognostic role of clinical, pathological and biological characteristics in patients with locally advanced breast cancer. Br J Cancer 1998;77:621–6.

53. Miller AB, Hoogstraten B, Staquet M, et al. Reporting results of cancer treatment. Cancer 1981;47:207–14.

54. Therasse P, Arbuck SG, Eisenhauer EA, et al. New guidelines to evaluate the response to treatment in solid tumors. J Natl Cancer Inst 2000;92:205–16.

55. Hamaoka T, Madewell JE, Podoloff DA, et al. Bone imaging in metastatic breast cancer. J Clin Oncol 2004;22:2942–53.

56. Price P, Jones T. Can positron emission tomography (PET) be used to detect subclinical response to cancer therapy? The EC PET Oncology Concerted Action and the EORTC PET Study Group. Eur J Cancer 1995;31A:1924–7.

57. Doot RK, Dunnwald LK, Schubert EK, et al. Dynamic and static approaches to quantifying 18F-FDG uptake for measuring cancer response to therapy, including the effect of granulocyte CSF. J Nucl Med 2007;48:920–5.

58. McIntosh SA, Ogston KN, Payne S, et al. Local recurrence in patients with large and locally advanced breast cancer treated with primary chemotherapy. Am J Surg 2003;185:525–31.

59. Beenken SW, Urist MM, Zhang Y, et al. Axillary lymph node status, but not tumor size, predicts locoregional recurrence and overall survival after mastectomy for breast cancer. Ann Surg 2003;237:732–9.

60. Burcombe RJ, Makris A, Pittam M, et al. Evaluation of good clinical response to neoadjuvant chemotherapy in primary breast cancer using [18F]-fluorodeoxyglucose positron emission tomography. Eur J Cancer 2002;38:375–9.

61. Mankoff DA, Dunnwald LK. Changes in glucose metabolism and blood flow following chemotherapy for breast cancer. PET Clin 2006;1:71–81.

62. Chen X, Moore MO, Lehman CD, et al. Combined use of MRI and PET to monitor response and assess residual disease for locally advanced breast cancer treated with neoadjuvant chemotherapy. Acad Radiol 2004;11:1115–24.

63. Solomayer EF, Diel IJ, Meyberg GC, et al. Metastatic breast cancer: clinical course, prognosis, and therapy related to the first site of metastasis. Breast Cancer Res Treat 2000;59(3):271–8.

64. Couturier O, Jerusalem G, N'Guyen JM, et al. Sequential positron emission tomography using [18F]fluorodeoxyglucose for monitoring response to chemotherapy in metastatic breast cancer. Clin Cancer Res 2006;12:6437–43.

65. Dose Schwarz J, Bader M, Jenicke L, et al. Early prediction of response to chemotherapy in metastatic breast cancer using sequential 18F-FDG PET. J Nucl Med 2005;46:1144–50.

66. Genarri A, Donati S, Salvadori B, et al. Role of 2-[18F] fluorodeoxyglucose (FDG) positron emission tomography (PET) in early assessment of response to

chemotherapy in metastatic breast cancer patients. Clin Breast Cancer 2000;1(2):156–61 [discussion: 162–3].

67. DeGiorgi U, Valero V, Rohren E, et al. Circulating tumor cells and [18F] fluorodeoxyglucose positron emission tomography/computed tomography for outcome prediction in metastatic breast cancer. J Clin Oncol 2009;27(20):3303–11.

68. Sagar SM, Klassen GA, Barclay KD, et al. Antitumor treatment: tumor blood flow—measurement and manipulation for therapeutic gain. Cancer Treat Rev 1993;19:299–349.

69. Mankoff DA, Dunnwald LK, Gralow JR, et al. Monitoring the response of patients with locally advanced breast carcinoma to neoadjuvant chemotherapy using [technetium-99m]-sestamibi scintimammography. Cancer 1999;85:2410–23.

70. Wilson CB, Lammertsma AA, McKenzie CG, et al. Measurements of blood flow and exchanging water space in breast tumors using positron emission tomography: a rapid and non-invasive dynamic method. Cancer Res 1992;52:1592–7.

71. Teicher BA. Hypoxia and drug resistance. Cancer Metastasis Rev 1994;13:139–68.

72. Mullani NA, Herbst RS, O'Neil RG, et al. Tumor blood flow measured by PET dynamic imaging of first-pass 18F-FDG uptake: a comparison with 15O-labeled water-measured blood flow. J Nucl Med 2008;49: 517–23.

73. Tseng J, Dunnwald LK, Schubert EK, et al. 18F-FDG kinetics in locally advanced breast cancer: correlation with tumor blood flow and changes in response to neoadjuvant chemotherapy. J Nucl Med 2004;45: 1829–37.

74. Zasadny KR, Tatsumi M, Wahl RL. FDG metabolism and uptake versus blood flow in women with untreated primary breast cancers. Eur J Nucl Med Mol Imaging 2003;30:274–80.

75. Katzenellenbogen JA. Designing steroid receptor-based radiotracers to image breast and prostate tumors. J Nucl Med 1995;36(6 Suppl):8S–13S.

76. Harris L, Fritsche H, Mennel R, et al. American Society of Clinical Oncology 2007 update of recommendations for the use of tumor markers in breast cancer. J Clin Oncol 2007;25:5287–312.

77. Smith-Jones PM, Solit D, Afroze F, et al. Early tumor response to Hsp90 therapy using HER2 PET: comparison with 18F-FDG PET. J Nucl Med 2006;47:793–6.

78. Specht JM, Tam SL, Kurland BF, et al. Serial 2-[18F] fluoro-2-deoxy-D-glucose positron emission tomography (FDG-PET) to monitor treatment of bone-dominant metastatic breast cancer predicts time to progression (TTP). Breast Cancer Res Treat 2007; 105:87–94.

Breast Cancer Imaging with Novel PET Tracers

David A. Mankoff, MD, PhD[a],*, Jean H. Lee, MD[b],
William B. Eubank, MD[c]

KEYWORDS

- PET • PET/CT • Breast cancer • Imaging
- Biomarker • Response

As the array of available treatments for breast cancer increases and therapy is increasingly targeted and individualized, there is an increasing need for information that can help direct therapy.[1-3] The imaging approaches in current clinical use for diagnosing and staging breast cancer—mammography, ultrasound, contrast-enhanced Magnetic resonance (MR) imaging, computed tomography (CT), bone scan, and ^{18}F-fluorodeoxyglucose (FDG)-PET/CT—provide important information on disease extent and response to treatment, but are relatively nonspecific.[4-6] PET radiopharmaceuticals beyond FDG can provide information about in vivo breast cancer biology from phenotype to early treatment response.[7] Novel tracers for PET breast cancer imaging will likely be used as cancer biomarkers, helping to direct therapeutic choices.[8,9] Specific and quantitative imaging approaches will be needed.

This article highlights examples of novel PET imaging approaches and radiopharmaceuticals that have undergone early studies in patients but are not approved for, or routinely used in, clinical practice. These approaches include measurement of tumor perfusion and angiogenesis, drug delivery and transport, tumor receptor expression, and early response to treatment.

TUMOR PERFUSION

Tumor vasculature is important in the development of invasive cancer, metastasis, and progression, and in the systemic delivery of therapeutic agents.[10] In addition, it is increasingly a target of anticancer therapy.[1] Antiangiogenic agents such as bevacizumab are now used as part of Food and Drug Administration (FDA)-approved breast cancer treatments.[11] Imaging tumor perfusion and neovasculature is a clinical important need.[12] Although many modalities, for example, contrast-enhanced CT, image tumor perfusion indirectly, the most physiologically robust and quantitative measures of tumor blood flow using freely diffusible imaging probes. For this class of imaging agents, blood flow can be inferred from the time course of uptake and washout, adapting methods developed for measuring cerebral blood flow.[13] For breast cancer, ^{15}O-water PET has been used to measure tumor blood flow. This method produces estimates of tumor blood flow in milliliters per minute per gram, and has been shown to yield reliable and reproducible estimates of tumor blood flow for breast cancer and other tumors.[14,15] Measuring change in tumor perfusion can be a very effective means of predicting response to systemic therapy for breast cancer.

This work was supported in part by NIH grants RO1CA42045, RO1CA72064, RO1CA124573, and S10RR177229.
[a] Department of Radiology, University of Washington and Seattle Cancer Care Alliance, G2-600, 825 Eastlake Avenue East, Seattle, WA 98109, USA
[b] Department of Radiology, University of Washington Medical Center, University of Washington and Seattle Cancer Care Alliance, Box 357115, Room BB308, 959 NE Pacific Street, Seattle, WA 98195, USA
[c] Department of Radiology (S-114-RAD), Puget Sound VA Health Care System, 1660 South Columbian Way, Seattle, WA 98108-1597, USA
* Corresponding author. Department of Radiology, University of Washington and Seattle Cancer Care Alliance, G2-600, 825 Eastlake Avenue East, Seattle, WA 98109.
E-mail address: dam@u.washington.edu (D.A. Mankoff).

PET Clin 4 (2009) 371–380
doi:10.1016/j.cpet.2009.10.003

Recent studies have shown that serial measures of breast cancer perfusion by water PET in the neo-adjuvant setting are highly predictive of response and survival.[16,17]

Some studies have also suggested that dynamic FDG-PET imaging and kinetic analysis may provide measures of tumor perfusion comparable to those from ^{15}O-water PET, inferred from the FDG delivery (K_1) kinetic parameter.[18–20] Other studies have shown that FDG K_1 correlates with other imaging measures of breast cancer perfusion, for example, estimates from dynamic contrast-enhanced MR imaging.[21] Recent studies have suggested that changes in FDG K_1 with chemotherapy are comparably predictive of response and survival.[17] Thus it may be possible to obtain information on both tumor perfusion and metabolism that is clinically predictive from dynamic FDG-PET. This approach merits further investigation.

Although perfusion imaging measures the physiologic consequences of angiogenesis, perfusion is not specific to tumor neovessels, and is influenced by physiologic parameters not necessarily related to tumor angiogenesis.[10] Targeted imaging probes can noninvasively and specifically assess tumor neovasculature.[22,23] PET probes based on specific labeled peptides that bind to integrins expressed in neovessels have been studied in animals and tested in humans,[24] including breast cancer patients.[25] The recent study of Beer and colleagues[25] showed uptake of ^{18}F-galacto-RGD, a probe directed at integrin expression in tumor neovasculature, in both primary and metastatic breast cancer. Another study using a slightly different compound, ^{18}F-AH111585, also targeted to integrins, showed similarly promising results.[26] Comparison with in vitro assay for integrin expression suggested that uptake reflected integrin expression in the tumor vasculature. Imaging agents targeted to neovessels, such as bevacizumab, may be especially helpful for therapies directed at tumor neovasculature.

The combination of tumor perfusion and metabolism imaging may yield further insights. Unlike normal tissues, there is considerable variation in the relationship between breast cancer metabolism and perfusion measured by FDG and water PET, or by PET and MR imaging.[19,20,27–29] Studies have shown that the relationship between metabolism and perfusion is predictive of therapeutic response and patient outcome.[17,28,29] An imbalance between metabolism and perfusion, indicated by high metabolism relative to perfusion (**Fig. 1**), is associated with poor response and early relapse.[17] A similar phenomenon has been found in other tumors,[30] and may be related to

fundamental cell survival mechanisms also seen in normal tissue such as the myocardium.[31,32] Further study of the biologic mechanism underlying these findings may yield insight into these striking results.

DRUG DELIVERY AND TRANSPORT

Effective cancer treatment by systemic therapy requires delivery and retention of the therapeutic agent at cancer sites. PET imaging provides a potentially powerful tool to determine drug pharmacokinetics, transport, and metabolism, with the goal of optimizing drug development and clinical use.[33–35] Several agents and approaches have been developed for this purpose; here some work of relevance to breast cancer treatment is highlighted.

Drug transporters are key in determining the clearance of cancer drugs from the body and also in mediating delivery to the tumor. Transporters, for example, nucleoside transporters, may mediate drug delivery into cancer cells. Other transporters, for example, drug efflux transporters such as P-glycoprotein (P-gp), may transport drugs out of cancer cells and thereby mediate drug resistance.[36] Considerable attention has been devoted to the imaging of drug efflux by P-gp in breast cancer.[37] Many of the chemotherapy agents that are important for breast cancer, such as doxorubicin, taxanes, and vinca alkaloids, are substrates for P-gp. It has been hypothesized that P-gp expression by tumors leads to resistance to these agents. Early studies focused on ^{99m}Tc-sestamibi (MIBI), based on the finding that MIBI is also a substrate for P-gp.[38] Studies showed that MIBI efflux rates correlated with P-gp expression in breast cancer and that a high rate of MIBI washout predicted poor response to treatment.[39–41] However, not all studies agree on the predictive value of MIBI washout,[42] and dependence of MIBI uptake and washout on tumor blood flow may confound interpretation of MIBI in vivo kinetics.[43]

Problems in the interpretation of MIBI images to estimate P-gp function, and the desire for more quantitative rigor, led to the development of PET P-gp imaging probes.[44] One of the most widely tested is ^{11}C-verapamil.[45] Verapamil is a well-validated P-gp substrate, and the kinetics of ^{11}C-verapamil reflect P-gp function.[46] Quantitative analysis of ^{11}C-verapamil kinetics provides a quantitative measure of P-gp function.[45] The short half-life of ^{11}C allows paired imaging studies with and without P-gp inhibition to measure directly the effect of P-gp on drug transport.[47,48] This approach provides an attractive method for testing

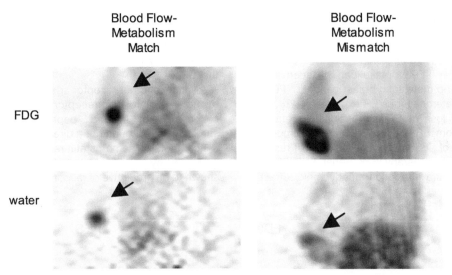

Fig. 1. Blood-flow metabolism mismatch imaged by PET. Sagittal summed images of FDG retention (*top*) and water delivery (*bottom*) are shown for 2 patients with locally advanced breast cancer. Images show that the patient in the left column had a quantitatively and regionally matched metabolism and blood flow, whereas the patient on the right has both quantitative and regional mismatches. The patient on the left had a pathologic complete response to neoadjuvant chemotherapy, whereas the patient on the right had significant residual viable tumor at postchemotherapy surgery.

the extent to which of P-gp limits drug uptake in tumors.

Investigators have also studied P-gp function using labeled taxanes, most notably ^{18}F-labeled fluoropaclitaxel.[49–52] Because taxanes are widely used in breast cancer, the retention of fluoropaclitaxel has direct relevance to breast cancer therapy. Some studies have suggested that uptake of fluoropaclitaxel may provide a direct prediction of the efficacy of therapeutic paclitaxel.[51] This approach has also been extended to other chemotherapy agents used in breast cancer, including cyclophosphamide and capecitibine.[53,54]

TUMOR RECEPTOR IMAGING

The ability to measure the expression of specific gene products associated with breast cancer has led to important advances in breast cancer treatment. The ability to image tumor receptors is particularly relevant to breast cancer treatment, and includes the expression of estrogen receptors (ERs), a target for endocrine therapy,[55] and HER2, also increasingly a target of tumor-specific treatment.[56] Tumor receptors are typically measured by in vitro assay of biopsy material.[57] Advantages of imaging for receptor expression measurement include its noninvasiveness, the ability to measure receptor expression in the entire disease burden and thus the ability to avoid sampling error that can occur with heterogeneous receptor

expression, and the potential for serial studies of in vivo drug effects on the target.[58] These advantages make tumor receptor imaging a complementary approach to in vitro assay of biopsy material. A practical consideration is that imaging can assess receptor expression at sites that are challenging to sample and assay, for example, bone metastases, whereby the need for tissue decalcification can make the assay of tumor gene products challenging.

Imaging tumor receptors poses some unique challenges not encountered in other areas of PET cancer imaging.[58] Small quantities of the imaging agent may saturate the receptor, and limit the ability to image and measure receptor expression.[59,60] For this reason, molecular imaging of tumor receptors has been most successful to date with radionuclide imaging, PET, and single photon emission CT (SPECT), whereby it is possible to generate images with nanomolar or picomolar amounts of the imaging probe.

Most work to date for breast cancer tumor receptor imaging has been done for steroid receptors.[58,61] Considerable efforts have gone into the development of radiopharmaceuticals for ER imaging, as reviewed by Mankoff and colleagues[58] and Katzenellenbogen.[61] The most successful ER imaging radiopharmaceutical to date is 16α-[^{18}F]fluoro-17β-estradiol (FES).[60] This agent can be synthesized with sufficient specific activity such that high-quality images of patients can be made with injections of less than 5 μg of FES.

Regional estrogen binding can be measured by FES-PET, and FES uptake has been validated as a measure of ER expression in breast tumors against ER expression assay of tissue samples.[62,63] FES uptake can be seen in both primary and metastatic breast cancer.[64] FES can identify heterogeneous ER expression (**Fig. 2**), for example, loss of ER expression in metastases arising from ER-expressing primary tumors.[64,65] The level of FES uptake is predictive of response to endocrine therapy.[65,66] Serial FES-PET can also measure the pharmacodynamic effect of

drugs on estradiol binding to the ER, yielding insights into determinants of drug efficacy.[58] Ongoing trials with this agent look promising, and this may be a tracer for use in the clinic in the future.

A variety of other receptor agents has also been tested.[58] Somatostatin receptor imaging of breast cancer using labeled peptides has been studied.[67,68] Although not a direct target or breast cancer therapy, somatostatin receptor expression measured by uptake of labeled probes has been shown to be predictive of response to ER-directed

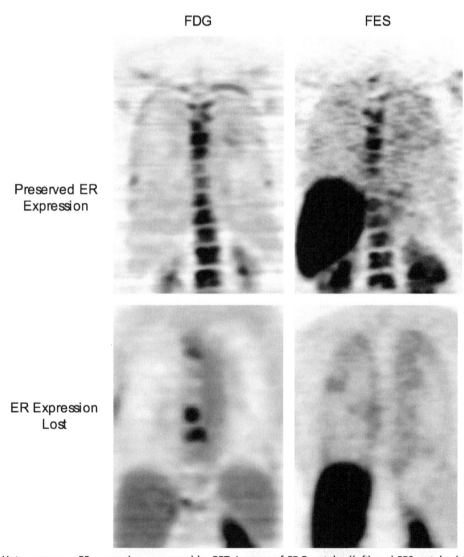

Fig. 2. Heterogeneous ER expression measured by PET. Images of FDG uptake (*left*) and FES uptake (*right*) are shown for 2 patients with bone metastases from ER-expressing primary tumors. The top patient has FES uptake at all sites of extensive abnormal FDG uptake, indicating preserved ER expression. The bottom patient has no FES uptake at sites of active disease seen by FDG-PET, indicating loss of ER expression in the metastases. Uptake in liver and kidneys, a normal finding related to modes of FES metabolism and excretion, is seen in both patients' FES PET images.

therapy.[68] Sigma receptor imaging has also been developed,[69–71] and may also be helpful in measuring tumor proliferation.[72]

HER2 (ErbB2) expression is an indicator of prognosis in breast cancer and an increasingly important target for therapy.[73] PET imaging approaches for measuring regional HER2 expression in breast cancer have also been developed. Most studies to date have used imaging probes based on immune recognition to image HER2 expression. Specific imaging probes based on radiolabeled antibodies, fragments, or novel constructs such as affibodies, have shown success in early studies (reviewed by Mankoff and colleagues[58]). Studies using a ^{68}Ga-labeled F(ab')$_2$ fragment of trastuzumab by Smith-Jones and colleagues[74] demonstrated the feasibility of measuring regional HER2 expression in murine animal models. The imaging results demonstrated an early decrease in HER2 expression accompanying experimental therapy using HSP90-directed agents (geldamycin analogues) to disrupt protein chaperoning, thereby reducing HER2 expression.[74] Studies using [131]I- or ^{111}In-labeled trastuzumab have demonstrated the ability to image tumor expression of HER2 and tumor and normal tissue, and to measure accumulation of trastuzumab,[75,76] although there has been some controversy about the significance of uptake in normal tissues prone to trastuzumab toxicity, such as the heart.[75,76] There have been promising early patient studies imaging HER2 expression by PET imaging using [89]Zr-labeled trastuzumab.[77]

IMAGING OF EARLY RESPONSE

Studies of FDG-PET in breast cancer chemotherapy have shown its ability to measure changes in uptake early in the course of treatment.[78–80] However, it is likely that other pathways more closely tied to cellular growth and death than glucose metabolism can provide even earlier and more specific measures of response.

Several methods have addressed tumor biosynthesis as an indicator of tumor growth, and have targeted protein synthesis and membrane synthesis. Labeled amino acids, such as ^{11}C-methionine, have been shown to provide an early indication of breast cancer response to therapy.[81] This approach, however, is limited by the complex nature of amino acid metabolism pathways, making it difficult to interpret uptake as measuring biosynthesis, versus amino acid transport and metabolism.[82]

Proliferating tumor cells also engage in enhanced lipid biosynthesis to provide cellular membranes needed for cell growth and division.[83] This process has been imaged by magnetic resonance spectroscopy,[84,85] largely examining choline concentration, and by PET, using labeled choline or acetate derivatives. Changes in the choline concentration measured by MR spectroscopy early in treatment seem to be a marker for early response to therapy, as early as 24 hours after treatment with chemotherapy.[86] Lipid metabolism is studied by PET using either [11]C- or ^{18}F-labeled choline, or ^{11}C-acetate,[87] which enters lipid synthesis pathways from the TCA cycle via fatty acid synthetase (FAS). FAS has been shown to have increased activity and expression in cancer and may be a target for therapy.[88] This approach has shown considerable promise in other tumors such as prostate cancer,[89] including therapeutic response,[90] but has had only limited testing in breast cancer.[91]

Aberrant cellular proliferation is a fundamental property of cancer[92] and provides an attractive means of evaluating response to treatment. Labeled compounds such as [14]C- or ^{3}H-thmyidine have constituted an important laboratory method for measuring cellular proliferation for more than 40 years.[93] Other methods of in vitro cellular proliferation assay, typically measuring MIB-1 (Ki-67) expresson,[94] are routinely performed in many centers as part of clinical care. Early work using ^{11}C-thymidine to measure tumor proliferation by PET were validated against in vitro assay gold standards and underwent preliminary testing in patients.[95] However, the short half-life of [11]C (20 minutes) and in vivo metabolism of thymidine provided important practical hurdles for this approach in clinical patient imaging. More recent work using thymidine analogs labeled with [18]F (half-life 109 minutes) have been developed and have undergone considerable advances in recent years.[95,96] The most promising of these is ^{18}F-fluorothymidine (FLT). Recent results in both animal and patient studies have demonstrated the potential utility of FLT-PET for breast cancer imaging.[97–100] FLT-PET's greatest promise for breast cancer lies in early response assessment, as suggested by recent studies of Pio and colleagues[99] and Kenny and colleagues.[98] These studies showed that serial FLT-PET could separate responders and nonresponders as early as one cycle after chemotherapy. FLT-PET is an exciting area of imaging research and is likely to be of clinical importance in the future. Clinical trials of FLT in breast cancer will be opening in the near future to much anticipation.

Cell death or apoptosis is a fundamental part of normal cellular physiology, and may also provide an early indicator of therapeutic response.[101] Methods for imaging cell death have been investigated. Many of these have been based on an extension of Annexin V staining in vitro, which indicates apoptotic cells through binding to phosphatidylserines.[102] The molecules are found only on the inner surface of plasma membranes and therefore are normally not accessible to Annexin V, a peptide, for binding. However, during apoptosis these molecules are transiently exposed to the extracellular space, allowing binding of Annexin.[102] The earliest studies used ^{99m}Tc-annexin and SPECT imaging to measure apoptosis in animal models and patients.[102,103] More recently, methods for Annexin-based apoptosis imaging have been developed for PET.[104,105] One limitation of this approach has been the transient nature of phosphatidylserine exposure during cell death, resulting in fairly limited signals for imaging.[106] Other approaches targeted to other aspects of the apoptotic cascade are being investigated.[104]

SUMMARY

PET imaging with tracers beyond FDG hold great promise for helping to guide individualized breast cancer therapy. Notable early studies in patients with breast carcinoma of imaging of tumor perfusion, specific imaging of tumor vasculature, drug transport, tumor receptors, and tumor proliferation provide an enticing and exciting glimpse of future direction for PET breast cancer imaging. Further preclinical development is ongoing and early clinical trials are underway. In the future, these novel PET tracers will very likely add to current capabilities with FDG PET, and improve the approach to clinical breast diagnostic and treatment selection.

REFERENCES

1. Doyle DM, Miller KD. Development of new targeted therapies for breast cancer. Breast Cancer 2008; 15(1):49–56.
2. Kaklamani V, O'Regan RM. New targeted therapies in breast cancer. Semin Oncol 2004;31(2 Suppl 4): 20–5.
3. Olopade OI, Grushko TA, Nanda R, et al. Advances in breast cancer: pathways to personalized medicine. Clin Cancer Res 2008;14(24):7988–99.
4. Benard F, Turcotte E. Imaging in breast cancer: Single-photon computed tomography and positron-emission tomography. Breast Cancer Res 2005;7(4):153–62.
5. Lee JH, Rosen EL, Mankoff DA. The role of radiotracer imaging in the diagnosis and management of patients with breast cancer: part 1—overview, detection, and staging. J Nucl Med 2009;50: 569–81.
6. Lee JH, Rosen EL, Mankoff DA. The role of radiotracer imaging in the diagnosis and management of patients with breast cancer: part 2—response to therapy, other indications, and future directions. J Nucl Med 2009;50(5):738–48.
7. Kelloff GJ, Krohn KA, Larson SM, et al. The progress and promise of molecular imaging probes in oncologic drug development. Clin Cancer Res 2005;11(22):7967–85.
8. Mankoff DA, O'Sullivan F, Barlow WE, et al. Molecular imaging research in the outcomes era: measuring outcomes for individualized cancer therapy. Acad Radiol 2007;14(4):398–405.
9. Weber WA. Positron emission tomography as an imaging biomarker. J Clin Oncol 2006;24(20): 3282–92.
10. Jain RK. Antiangiogenic therapy for cancer: current and emerging concepts. Oncology (Williston Park) 2005;19(4 Suppl 3):7–16.
11. Hayes DF, Miller K, Sledge G. Angiogenesis as targeted breast cancer therapy. Breast 2007; 16(Suppl 2):S17–9.
12. Miller JC, Pien HH, Sahani D, et al. Imaging angiogenesis: applications and potential for drug development. J Natl Cancer Inst 2005; 97(3):172–87.
13. Kety SS. Basic principles for the quantitative estimation of regional cerebral blood flow. Res Publ Assoc Res Nerv Ment Dis 1985;63:1–7.
14. Wilson CB, Lammertsma AA, McKenzie CG, et al. Measurements of blood flow and exchanging water space in breast tumors using positron emission tomography: a rapid and non-invasive dynamic method. Cancer Res 1992;52:1592–7.
15. Wells P, Jones T, Price P. Assessment of inter-inter and intrapatient variability in C[15]O$_2$ positron emission tomography measurements of blood flow in patients with intra-abdominal cancers. Clin Cancer Res 2003;9(17):6350–6.
16. Mankoff DA, Dunnwald LK, Gralow JR, et al. Changes in blood flow and metabolism in locally advanced breast cancer treated with neoadjuvant chemotherapy. J Nucl Med 2003;44(11):1806–14.
17. Dunnwald LK, Gralow JR, Ellis GK, et al. Tumor metabolism and blood flow changes by positron emission tomography: relation to survival in patients treated with neoadjuvant chemotherapy for locally advanced breast cancer. J Clin Oncol 2008;26(27):4449–5726.
18. Mullani NA, Herbst RS, O'Neil RG, et al. Tumor blood flow measured by PET dynamic imaging of first-pass ^{18}F-FDG uptake: a comparison with ^{15}O-labeled water-measured blood flow. J Nucl Med 2008;49(4):517–23.
19. Tseng J, Dunnwald LK, Schubert EK, et al. ^{18}F-FDG kinetics in locally advanced breast cancer: correlation with tumor blood flow and changes in response

to neoadjuvant chemotherapy. J Nucl Med 2004; 45(11):1829–37.

20. Zasadny KR, Tatsumi M, Wahl RL. FDG metabolism and uptake versus blood flow in women with untreated primary breast cancers. Eur J Nucl Med Mol Imaging 2003;30(2):274–80.

21. Eby PR, Partridge SC, White SW, et al. Metabolic and vascular features of dynamic contrast-enhanced breast magnetic resonance imaging and (15)O-water positron emission tomography blood flow in breast cancer. Acad Radiol 2008; 15(10):1246–54.

22. Schirner M, Menrad A, Stephens A, et al. Molecular imaging of tumor angiogenesis. Ann N Y Acad Sci 2004;1014:67–75.

23. Charnley N, Donaldson S, Price P. Imaging angiogenesis. Methods Mol Biol 2009;467:25–51.

24. Beer AJ, Haubner R, Sarbia M, et al. Positron emission tomography using [18F]Galacto-RGD identifies the level of integrin alpha(v)beta3 expression in man. Clin Cancer Res 2006;12(13):3942–9.

25. Beer AJ, Niemeyer M, Carlsen J, et al. Patterns of alphavbeta3 expression in primary and metastatic human breast cancer as shown by 18F-Galacto-RGD PET. J Nucl Med 2008;49(2):255–9.

26. Kenny LM, Coombes RC, Oulie I, et al. Phase I trial of the positron-emitting Arg-Gly-Asp (RGD) peptide radioligand 18F-AH111585 in breast cancer patients. J Nucl Med 2008;49(6):879–86.

27. Hentschel M, Paulus T, Mix M, et al. Analysis of blood flow and glucose metabolism in mammary carcinomas and normal breast: a H2(15)O PET and 18F-FDG PET study. Nucl Med Commun 2007;28(10):789–97.

28. Mankoff DA, Dunnwald LK, Gralow JR, et al. Blood flow and metabolism in locally advanced breast cancer: relationship to response to therapy. J Nucl Med 2002;43(4):500–9.

29. Semple SI, Gilbert FJ, Redpath TW, et al. The relationship between vascular and metabolic characteristics of primary breast tumours. Eur Radiol 2004;14(11):2038–45.

30. Miles KA, Williams RE. Warburg revisited: imaging tumour blood flow and metabolism. Cancer Imaging 2008;8:81–6.

31. Mankoff DA, Dunnwald LK, Partridge SC, et al. Blood flow-metabolism mismatch: good for the tumor, bad for the patient. Clin Cancer Res 2009; 15(17):5294–6.

32. Schelbert HR. PET contributions to understanding normal and abnormal cardiac perfusion and metabolism. Ann Biomed Eng 2000;28(8):922–9.

33. Aboagye EO, Price PM. Use of positron emission tomography in anticancer drug development. Invest New Drugs 2003;21(2):169–81.

34. Saleem A, Aboagye EO, Matthews JC, et al. Plasma pharmacokinetic evaluation of cytotoxic agents radiolabelled with positron emitting radioisotopes. Cancer Chemother Pharmacol 2008; 61(5):865–73.

35. Aboagye EO, Price PM, Jones T. In vivo pharmacokinetics and pharmacodynamics in drug development using positron-emission tomography. Drug Discov Today 2001;6(6):293–302.

36. Kaye SB. Multidrug resistance: clinical relevance in solid tumours and strategies for circumvention. Curr Opin Oncol 1998;10(Suppl 1):S15–9.

37. Fojo T, Coley HM. The role of efflux pumps in drug-resistant metastatic breast cancer: new insights and treatment strategies. Clin Breast Cancer 2007;7(10):749–56.

38. Piwnica-Worms D, Chiu ML, Budding M, et al. Functional imaging of multidrug-resistant P-glycoprotein with an organotechnetium complex. Cancer Res 1993;53(5):977–84.

39. Ciarmiello A, Vecchio SD, Silvestro P, et al. Tumor clearance of technetium 99m-sestamibi as a predictor of response to neoadjuvant chemotherapy for locally advanced breast cancer. J Clin Oncol 1998;16(5):1677–83.

40. Kostakoglu L, Ruacan S, Ergun EL, et al. Influence of the heterogeneity of P-glycoprotein expression on technetium-99m-MIBI uptake in breast cancer. J Nucl Med 1998;39(6):1021–6.

41. Sciuto R, Pasqualoni R, Bergomi S, et al. Prognostic value of (99m)Tc-sestamibi washout in predicting response of locally advanced breast cancer to neoadjuvant chemotherapy. J Nucl Med 2002;43(6):745–51.

42. Travaini LL, Baio SM, Cremonesi M, et al. Neoadjuvant therapy in locally advanced breast cancer: 99mTc-MIBI mammoscintigraphy is not a reliable technique to predict therapy response. Breast 2007;16(3):262–70.

43. Mankoff DA, Dunnwald LK, Gralow JR, et al. [Tc-99m]-sestamibi uptake and washout in locally advanced breast cancer are correlated with tumor blood flow. Nucl Med Biol 2002;29(7): 719–27.

44. Elsinga PH, Hendrikse NH, Bart J, et al. PET Studies on P-glycoprotein function in the blood-brain barrier: how it affects uptake and binding of drugs within the CNS. Curr Pharm Des 2004; 10(13):1493–503.

45. Hendrikse NH, de Vries EG, Eriks-Fluks L, et al. A new in vivo method to study P-glycoprotein transport in tumors and the blood-brain barrier. Cancer Res 1999;59(10):2411–6.

46. Hendrikse NH, de Vries EG, Franssen EJ, et al. In vivo measurement of [11C]verapamil kinetics in human tissues. Eur J Clin Pharmacol 2001;56(11): 827–9.

47. Sasongko L, Link JM, Muzi M, et al. Imaging P-glycoprotein transport activity at the human

blood-brain barrier with positron emission tomography. Clin Pharmacol Ther 2005;77(6):503–14.

48. Muzi M, Mankoff DA, Link JM, et al. Imaging of cyclosporine inhibition of P-glycoprotein activity using ^{11}C-verapamil in the brain: studies of healthy humans. J Nucl Med 2009;50(8):1267–75.

49. Kurdziel KA, Kalen JD, Hirsch JI, et al. Imaging multidrug resistance with 4-[^{18}F]fluoropaclitaxel. Nucl Med Biol 2007;34(7):823–31.

50. Kurziel KA, Kieswetter DO, Carson RE, et al. Biodistribution, radiation dose estimates, and in vivo P-gp modulation studies of ^{18}F-paclitaxel in nonhuman primates. J Nucl Med 2003;44:1330–9.

51. Hsueh WA, Kesner AL, Gangloff A, et al. Predicting chemotherapy response to paclitaxel with ^{18}F-Fluoropaclitaxel and PET. J Nucl Med 2006;47(12):1995–9.

52. Gangloff A, Hsueh WA, Kesner AL, et al. Estimation of paclitaxel biodistribution and uptake in human-derived xenografts in vivo with (18)F-fluoropaclitaxel. J Nucl Med 2005;46(11):1866–71.

53. Kesner AL, Hsueh WA, Htet NL, et al. Biodistribution and predictive value of ^{18}F-fluorocyclophosphamide in mice bearing human breast cancer xenografts. J Nucl Med 2007;48(12):2021–7.

54. Fei X, Wang JQ, Miller KD, et al. Synthesis of [^{18}F]Xeloda as a novel potential PET radiotracer for imaging enzymes in cancers. Nucl Med Biol 2004;31(8):1033–41.

55. Jordan VC, Brodie AM. Development and evolution of therapies targeted to the estrogen receptor for the treatment and prevention of breast cancer. Steroids 2007;72(1):7–25.

56. Slamon DJ, Leyland-Jones B, Shak S, et al. Use of chemotherapy plus a monoclonal antibody against HER2 for metastatic breast cancer that overexpresses HER2. N Engl J Med 2001;344(11):783–92.

57. Osborne CK, Yochmowitz MG, Knight WA 3rd, et al. The value of estrogen and progesterone receptors in the treatment of breast cancer. Cancer 1980;46(Suppl 12):2884–8.

58. Mankoff DA, Link JM, Linden HM, et al. Tumor receptor imaging. J Nucl Med 2008;49(Suppl 2):149S–63S.

59. Katzenellenbogen J. The pharmacology of steroid radiopharmaceuticals: specific and non-specific binding and uptake selectivity. In: Nunn A, editor. Radiopharmaceuticals: chemistry and pharmacology. New York: Marcel Dekker; 1992. p. 297–331.

60. Katzenellenbogen JA, Welch MJ, Dehdashti F. The development of estrogen and progestin radiopharmaceuticals for imaging breast cancer. Anticancer Res 1997;17:1573–6.

61. Katzenellenbogen JA. Designing steroid receptor-based radiotracers to image breast and prostate tumors. J Nucl Med 1995;36(Suppl 6):8S–13S.

62. Mintun MA, Welch MJ, Siegel BA, et al. Breast cancer: PET imaging of estrogen receptors. Radiology 1988;169(1):45–8.

63. Peterson LM, Mankoff DA, Lawton TJ, et al. Quantitative imaging of estrogen receptor expression of breast cancer with PET and [F-18'-fluorestradiol. J Nucl Med 2008;49(3):367–74.

64. Dehdashti F, Mortimer JE, Siegel BA, et al. Positron tomographic assessment of estrogen receptors in breast cancer: comparison with FDG-PET and in vitro receptor assays. J Nucl Med 1995;36(10):1766–74.

65. Linden HM, Stekhova SA, Link JM, et al. Quantitative fluoroestradiol positron emission tomography imaging predicts response to endocrine treatment in breast cancer. J Clin Oncol 2006;24(18):2793–9.

66. Mortimer JE, Dehdashti F, Siegel BA, et al. Metabolic flare: indicator of hormone responsiveness in advanced breast cancer. J Clin Oncol 2001;19(11):2797–803.

67. Mezi S, Primi F, Orsi E, et al. Somatostatin receptor scintigraphy in metastatic breast cancer patients. Oncol Rep 2005;13(1):31–5.

68. Van Den Bossche B, Van Belle S, De Winter F, et al. Early prediction of endocrine therapy effect in advanced breast cancer patients using 99mTc-depreotide scintigraphy. J Nucl Med 2006;47(1):6–13.

69. Tu Z, Xu J, Jones LA, et al. Fluorine-18-labeled benzamide analogues for imaging the sigma2 receptor status of solid tumors with positron emission tomography. J Med Chem 2007;50(14):3194–204.

70. Mach RH, Huang Y, Buchheimer N, et al. [(18)F]N-(4'-fluorobenzyl)-4-(3-bromophenyl) acetamide for imaging the sigma receptor status of tumors: comparison with [(18)F]FDG, and [(125)I]IUDR. Nucl Med Biol 2001;28(4):451–8.

71. Mach RH, Gage HD, Buchheimer N, et al. N-[^{18}F]4'-fluorobenzylpiperidin-4yl-(2-fluorophenyl) acetamide ([^{18}F]FBFPA): a potential fluorine-18 labeled PET radiotracer for imaging sigma-1 receptors in the CNS. Synapse 2005;58(4):267–74.

72. Wheeler KT, Wang LM, Wallen CA, et al. Sigma-2 receptors as a biomarker of proliferation in solid tumours. Br J Cancer 2000;82(6):1223–32.

73. Harris L, Fritsche H, Mennel R, et al. American Society of Clinical Oncology 2007 update of recommendations for the use of tumor markers in breast cancer. J Clin Oncol 2007;25(33):5287–312.

74. Smith-Jones PM, Solit D, Afroze F, et al. Early tumor response to Hsp90 therapy using HER2 PET: comparison with 18F-FDG PET. J Nucl Med 2006;47(5):793–6.

75. de Korte MA, de Vries EG, Lub-de Hooge MN, et al. (111)Indium-trastuzumab visualises myocardial human epidermal growth factor receptor 2 expression shortly after anthracycline treatment but not during heart failure: a clue to uncover the mechanisms of trastuzumab-related cardiotoxicity. Eur J Cancer 2007;43(14):2046–51.

76. Perik PJ, Lub-De Hooge MN, Gietema JA, et al. Indium-111-labeled trastuzumab scintigraphy in patients with human epidermal growth factor receptor 2-positive metastatic breast cancer. J Clin Oncol 2006;24(15):2276–82.

77. Dijkers EC, Kosterink JG, Rademaker AP, et al. Development and characterization of clinical-grade [89]Zr-trastuzumab for HER2/neu immunoPET imaging. J Nucl Med 2009;50(6):974–81.

78. Rousseau C, Devillers A, Sagan C, et al. Monitoring of early response to neoadjuvant chemotherapy in stage II and III breast cancer by [18F]fluorodeoxyglucose positron emission tomography. J Clin Oncol 2006;24(34):5366–72.

79. Schelling M, Avril N, Nahrig J, et al. Positron emission tomography using [18F] fluorodeoxyglucose for monitoring primary chemotherapy in breast cancer. J Clin Oncol 2000;18:1689–95.

80. Smith I, Welch A, Hutcheon A, et al. Positron emission tomography using [18F]-fluorodeoxy-D-glucose to predict the pathologic response of breast cancer to primary chemotherapy. J Clin Oncol 2000;18:1676–88.

81. Jansson T, Westlin JE, Ahlstrom H, et al. Positron emission tomography studies in patients with locally advanced and/or metastatic breast cancer: a method for early therapy evaluation? J Clin Oncol 1995;13(6):1470–7.

82. Ishiwata K, Enomoto K, Sasaki T, et al. A feasibility study on L-[1-carbon-11]tyrosine and L-[methyl-carbon-11]methionine to assess liver protein synthesis by PET. J Nucl Med 1996;37(2):279–85.

83. Glunde K, Jacobs MA, Bhujwalla ZM. Choline metabolism in cancer: implications for diagnosis and therapy. Expert Rev Mol Diagn 2006;6(6):821–9.

84. Bolan PJ, Nelson MT, Yee D, et al. Imaging in breast cancer: magnetic resonance spectroscopy. Breast Cancer Res 2005;7(4):149–52.

85. Stanwell P, Mountford C. In vivo proton MR spectroscopy of the breast. Radiographics 2007;27(Suppl 1):S253–66.

86. Meisamy S, Bolan PJ, Baker EH, et al. Neoadjuvant chemotherapy of locally advanced breast cancer: predicting response with in vivo (1)H MR spectroscopy—a pilot study at 4 T. Radiology 2004;233(2):424–31.

87. Groves AM, Win T, Haim SB, et al. Non-[18F]FDG PET in clinical oncology. Lancet Oncol 2007;8(9):822–30.

88. Lupu R, Menendez JA. Targeting fatty acid synthase in breast and endometrial cancer: an alternative to selective estrogen receptor modulators? Endocrinology 2006;147(9):4056–66.

89. Powles T, Murray I, Brock C, et al. Molecular positron emission tomography and PET/CT imaging in urological malignancies. Eur Urol 2007;51(6):1511–20 [discussion: 1520–1].

90. Yu EY, Mankoff DA. Positron emission tomography imaging as a cancer biomarker. Expert Rev Mol Diagn 2007;7(5):659–72.

91. Zheng QH, Stone KL, Mock BH, et al. [11C]Choline as a potential PET marker for imaging of breast cancer athymic mice. Nucl Med Biol 2002;29(8):803–7.

92. Tannock IF. Cell proliferation. In: Tannock IF, Hill RP, editors. The basic science of oncology. New York: McGraw-Hill; 1992. p. 154–77.

93. Cleaver JE. Thymidine metabolism and cell kinetics. Front Biol 1967;6:43–100.

94. Pinder SE, Wencyk P, Sibbering DM, et al. Assessment of the new proliferation marker MIB1 in breast carcinoma using image analysis: associations with other prognostic factors and survival. Br J Cancer 1995;71:146–9.

95. Mankoff DA, Shields AF, Krohn KA. PET imaging of cellular proliferation. Radiol Clin North Am 2005;43(1):153–67.

96. Shields AF, Grierson JR, Dohmen BM, et al. Imaging proliferation in vivo with [F-18]FLT and positron emission tomography. Nat Med 1998;4(11):1334–6.

97. Been LB, Elsinga PH, de Vries J, et al. Positron emission tomography in patients with breast cancer using (18)F-3′-deoxy-3′-fluoro-l-thymidine ((18)F-FLT)-a pilot study. Eur J Surg Oncol 2006;32(1):39–43.

98. Kenny L, Coombes RC, Vigushin DM, et al. Imaging early changes in proliferation at 1 week post chemotherapy: a pilot study in breast cancer patients with 3′-deoxy-3′-[18F]fluorothymidine positron emission tomography. Eur J Nucl Med Mol Imaging 2007;34(9):1339–47.

99. Pio BS, Park CK, Pietras R, et al. Usefulness of 3′-[F-18]fluoro-3′-deoxythymidine with positron emission tomography in predicting breast cancer response to therapy. Mol Imaging Biol 2006;8(1):36–42.

100. Smyczek-Gargya B, Fersis N, Dittmann H, et al. PET with [18F]fluorothymidine for imaging of primary breast cancer: a pilot study. Eur J Nucl Med Mol Imaging 2004;31(5):720–4.

101. Hockenbery D. Defining apoptosis. Am J Pathol 1995;146(1):16–9.

102. Blankenberg F, Ohtsuki K, Strauss HW. Dying a thousand deaths. Radionuclide imaging of apoptosis. Q J Nucl Med 1999;43(2):170–6.

103. van de Wiele C, Lahorte C, Vermeersch H, et al. Quantitative tumor apoptosis imaging using technetium-99m-HYNIC annexin V single photon emission computed tomography. J Clin Oncol 2003; 21(18):3483–7.

104. Schoenberger J, Bauer J, Moosbauer J, et al. Innovative strategies in in vivo apoptosis imaging. Curr Med Chem 2008;15(2):187–94.

105. Yagle KJ, Eary JF, Tait JF, et al. Evaluation of ^{18}F-annexin V as a PET imaging agent in an animal model of apoptosis. J Nucl Med 2005;46(4): 658–66.

106. Tait JF, Smith C, Blankenberg FG. Structural requirements for in vivo detection of cell death with 99mTc-annexin V. J Nucl Med 2005;46(5): 807–15.

Exploring Tumor Biology with Fluorodeoxyglucose–Positron Emission Tomography Imaging in Breast Carcinoma

Sandip Basu, MBBS (Hons), DRM, DNB, MNAMS[a],
Rakesh Kumar, MD[b], Ayşe Mavi, MD[c],
Abass Alavi, MD, MD (Hon), PhD (Hon), DSc (Hon)[d],*

KEYWORDS

- FDG-positron emission tomography
- Breast carcinoma • Triple-negative cancer

The value of fluorodeoxyglucose–positron emission tomography (FDG-PET)/computed tomography (CT) in breast carcinoma extends well beyond diagnostic staging and detection of primary lesions. An association between high FDG uptake and a worse prognosis has been emphasized in the recent literature. Several studies have been or are being performed correlating FDG uptake with various prognostic and molecular biomarkers as well as different parameters predicting tumor response to therapy. Innovative radiotracers for specific imaging of tumoral perfusion (eg, $[(15)O]H(2)O$), hormone receptor expression (eg, $[(18)F]FES$), protein synthesis (eg, $[(11)C]$methionine), and proliferation rate (eg, $[(18)F]FLT$) provide additional information about tumor characteristics and have been dealt with in detail by Mankoff and colleagues elsewhere in this issue.

In this article, the authors have classified the studies investigating FDG-PET imaging in depicting breast cancer biology into six different groups based upon the tumor characteristic that was correlated with the FDG uptake in the particular study. These are listed in **Box 1** and **Table 1**.

STUDIES INVESTIGATING FDG UPTAKE WITH TUMOR SUBTYPES

There has been significant evidence that FDG accumulation in breast cancer is primarily GLUT1-mediated and that the ductal carcinomas are more metabolically active that the lobular subtype (**Fig. 1**), commensurate with their known aggressive biology compared with the latter.

In the study by Buck and colleagues[1] that investigated FDG accumulation in primary breast cancer, FDG uptake was significantly higher in ductal carcinoma than in lobular carcinoma (mean tumor-to-background ratio, 17.3 vs 6.5, respectively). Of all the parameters examined in this study (c-erb B2, tumor grade, estrogen receptor [ER] status, progesterone receptor [PR] status, tumor size, axillary lymph node status, proliferation index, and Ki-67), only Ki-67 showed

a Radiation Medicine Centre (BARC), Tata Memorial Hospital Annexe, Parel, Mumbai, India
b Department of Nuclear Medicine, All India Institute of Medical Sciences, New Delhi, 110029, India
c Department of Nuclear Medicine, Yeditepe University Hospital, Istanbul, Turkey
d Nuclear Medicine Section, Radiology Department, Hospital of the University of Pennsylvania, Philadelphia, PA, USA
* Corresponding author.
E-mail address: abass.alavi@uphs.upenn.edu (A. Alavi).

PET Clin 4 (2009) 381–389
doi:10.1016/j.cpet.2009.12.001

Box 1
Classification of studies investigating breast carcinoma biology

Studies investigating FDG uptake with tumor subtypes

Studies investigating FDG uptake with hormonal receptor expression in the tumor

Studies investigating FDG uptake with disease burden at diagnosis

Studies investigating FDG uptake with tumor proliferation index and other parameters

Studies investigating the correlation of FDG uptake with that of other PET tracers

In vitro studies in breast cancer cell lines

a statistically significant positive correlation to FDG accumulation in ductal breast cancer. Similar results were obtained by Crippa and colleagues,[2] who showed that the tumor median SUV was significantly higher in the infiltrating ductal carcinomas than in the lobular carcinomas (5.6 vs 3.8, respectively) and higher in grade 3 carcinomas than in grade 1–2 carcinomas (6.2 vs 4.9, respectively).

STUDIES INVESTIGATING FDG UPTAKE WITH HORMONAL RECEPTOR EXPRESSION IN THE TUMOR

The authors' research[3] has suggested that breast cancer that lacks estrogen, progesterone, and Her-2/neu receptor expression, often known as triple-negative cancer, took up FDG more avidly than nontriple-negative breast cancer. In the study by Basu and colleagues,[3] newly diagnosed breast carcinoma patients, who had undergone dual time point FDG-PET before any therapeutic intervention and were found to be either ER–/PR–/HER2– or ER+/PR+/HER2– (the control group) on histopathology of the surgical specimen, were considered candidates for inclusion in this analysis. These patients underwent FDG-PET as a component of a prospective study evaluating the role of multimodality imaging for characterizing primary breast lesions and locoregional staging. Maximum standardized uptake values (SUVmax) were measured at both time points (SUVmax1 and SUVmax2) for the analysis of the data generated. Following FDG PET imaging, the patients underwent either breast-conserving surgery or mastectomy, and reports of histopathology were considered to provide the definitive diagnosis against which the PET study results were compared.

Eighty-eight patients with breast cancer (29 patients with triple-negative breast cancer and 59 patients with ER+/PR+/HER2 breast malignancy) were selected from 206 individuals who were enrolled in the study protocol. The triple-negative group comprised 14.08% of the total study population. The age of the patients with this subtype of tumor ranged from 33 to 75 years (mean 51.6 plus or minus 10.1 years), and the tumor size in this subgroup ranged from 0.9 to 6 cm (mean: 1.99 cm). Among the histopathological subtypes, 25 cases were infiltrating ductal carcinoma (86%), and 1 case was reported for each of the following (3.5% each subtype): lobular, mixed ductal–lobular, medullary, and tubular carcinomas. For the calculation of FDG-PET parameters in this group, the authors considered strictly those patients who had undergone FDG-PET studies before any intervention, and 18 patients in the triple-negative group met this criterion. Following the same criterion, a control group of 59 patients of ER+ve/PR+ve/HER2-ve cancer who had shown focal FDG uptake was selected for comparison with this population. The breast cancer lesions were visualized as areas with focally enhanced uptake of FDG in all the cases (sensitivity 100%) of the triple-negative group.

The mean SUVmax1 of the primary lesion of the triple negative group was 7.27 plus or minus 5.6; mean SUVmax2 was 8.29 plus or minus 6.4, and %ΔSUVmax was 14.3% plus or minus 15.8%. In 59 patients with ER+ve/PR+ve/HER2-ve breast carcinoma, the mean SUVmax1, SUVmax2, and the %ΔSUVmax were 2.68% plus or minus 1.9%, 2.84% plus or minus 2.2%, and 3.7% plus or minus 13.0%, respectively. The mean SUVmax1, SUVmax2, and %ΔSUVmax of triple negative cancer were significantly higher than those of the nontriple-negative control group ($P = .0032$, .002, and .017, respectively).

When the authors compared the two subgroups according to size, grade, and stage, they found that the SUVmax1 is significantly higher in triple-negative cancer for both size categories (5.4 vs 1.9, $P = .006$ and 9.2 vs 3.5, $P = .04$) and the grade 3 tumors (9.1 vs 3.9, $P = .022$). The ΔSUVmax in the triple-negative group below 2 cm and above 2 cm was 14.8 and 13.8, respectively. The corresponding figures for the ER+ve/PR+ve/HER2-ve group were 0.6 and 6.7, respectively. Although the mean ΔSUVmax was clearly higher in the triple-negative group in both tumor size categories, comparison between the two groups demonstrated a statistically significant difference in tumors with less than 2 cm ($P = .016$). The authors also observed that tumor grades of triple-negative cancer significantly correlated with the magnitude

Table 1
Important studies investigating the utility FDG-PET imaging in defining breast carcinoma biology

Authors	Year	Tumor Characteristic Investigated	Salient Findings of the Study
Buck et al	2002	Histologic subtypes and other factors	Ductal carcinomas are more metabolically active than the lobular subtype, and Ki-67 showed a statistically significant positive correlation to FDG accumulation in ductal breast cancer
Crippa et al	1998	Histologic subtypes and grade	Tumor median SUV was significantly higher in IDCs than the lobular carcinomas and in grade 3 carcinomas than in grade 1–2 carcinomas
Basu et al	2008	Hormonal receptor status	Triple-negative cancer concentrated FDGs more avidly commensurate with their aggressive biology and were detected with very high sensitivity by using FDG-PET imaging
Mavi et al	2007	Hormonal receptors	ER-positive tumors concentrate more FDG than ER-negative lesions, and interactions exist between ER and C-erbB-2R states and between PR and C-erbB-2R states
Basu et al	2008	Disease burden at diagnosis	Higher FDG accumulation can effectively reflect the metastatic propensity of the tumor
Avril et al	2000	Ki 67 status in the tumor	Significant correlation between FDG uptake and proliferation index
Shimoda et al	2007	Early and delayed phase mitotic counts, Ki67 positive cell percentage and nuclear grade	Significant association between FDG accumulation and early and delayed phase mitotic counts, Ki67 positive cell percentage and nuclear grade
Tchou et al	2009	Percent Ki67 nuclear stain of triple-negative breast cancer	Significant correlation noted in the subset of women with triple-negative cancer compared with the entire cohort
Bos et al	2002	Microvasculature density, GLUT1 and hexokinase expression, proliferation rate, number of lymphocytes, HIF-1a up-regulation of GLUT1, mitotic activity index (MAI), amount of necrosis	Significant correlation noted between FDG uptake and microvasculature density, GLUT1 and hexokinase expression, proliferation rate, number of lymphocytes, and HIF-1a up-regulation of GLUT1
Burgman et al	2001	GLUT activity in MCF-7 breast cancer cells	Hypoxia-induced increase in FDG accumulation in MCF-7 breast cancer cells is in part related to an increase in GLUT activity
Tseng et al	2004	Characterize and correlate the biologic response of locally advanced breast cancer (LABC) to chemotherapy using ^{15}O-water and ^{18}F-FDG-PET parameters	The pattern of tumor glucose metabolism in LABC, as reflected by analysis of FDG rate parameters, changes after therapy

Abbreviations: ER, estrogen receptor; IDC, infiltrating duct carcinoma; PR, progesterone receptor; SUV, standardized uptake value.

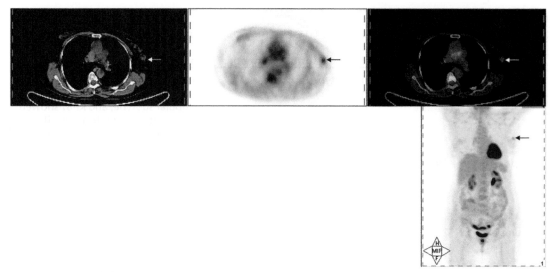

Fig. 1. A primary left breast lesion, diagnosed to be lobular left breast cancer having relatively low SUV (SUVmax: 1.2).

of SUVmax1 and SUVmax2 (*P* = .012 and .01, respectively). Stage for stage, triple-negative cancer appeared to have a higher mean SUVmax1 when compared with the nontriple-negative control group. The authors concluded that triple-negative breast cancer is associated with enhanced FDG uptake commensurate with its aggressive biology, and it is detected with very high sensitivity with FDG-PET imaging (**Figs. 2–4**).

In another study by Mavi and colleagues,[4] 213 patients with newly diagnosed breast cancer underwent 18F-FDG-PET to investigate whether correlations exist between 18F-FDG uptake of primary breast cancer lesions and predictive and prognostic factors such as ER, PR, and C-erbB-2 receptor (C-erbB-2R) state. The mean maximum SUVs of ER-positive and ER-negative lesions were 3.03 plus or minus 0.26 and 5.64 plus or minus 0.75, whereas those of PR were 3.24 plus or minus 0.29 and 4.89 plus or minus 0.67, respectively, and those of C-erbB-2R were 4.64 plus or minus 0.70 and 3.70 plus or minus 0.35, respectively. Chi2 tests for ER and PR showed that if one is positive then the other tends to be positive also (chi2 = 71.054, *P*<.01). For ER and C-erbB-2R states, if ER is positive, C-erbB-2R will more likely be negative (chi2 = 13.026, *P*<.01). The results demonstrated that interactions exist between ER and C-erbB-2R state and between PR and C-erbB-2R state.

STUDIES INVESTIGATING FDG UPTAKE WITH DISEASE BURDEN AT DIAGNOSIS

A study[5] that correlated the level of FDG uptake in the primary breast tumor with that of disease

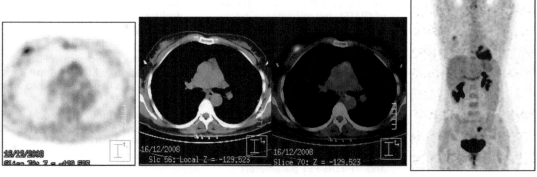

Fig. 2. Right breast ER-positive, PR-positive, cerb b2-negative invasive ductal carcinoma, tumor size: 4 × 3 cm, SUVmax1: 1.6, SUVmax2: 1.6 (no change).

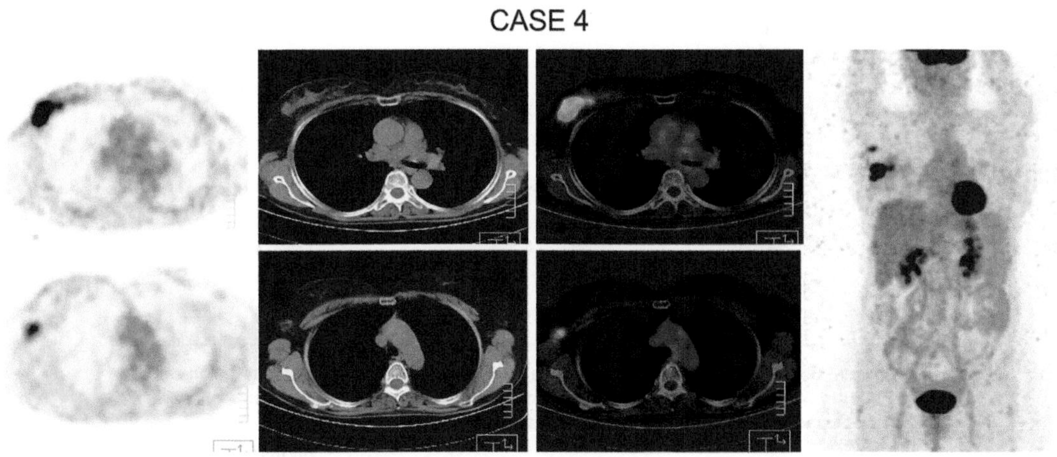

CASE 4

Fig. 3. Right breast invasive ductal carcinoma with axillary lymph node metastasis, receptor status: ER-negative, PR-negative, cerb b2-positive, SUVmax: 12.8, axillary node SUVmax: 4.4.

burden at diagnosis found that the uptake can be a good surrogate marker for the amount of expected disease burden both locally in the axilla and in distant sites. This study examined 174 patients with newly diagnosed breast cancer who were divided into three groups: 64 patients with primary and metastatic axillary lymphadenopathy (group 1), 18 patients with both axillary and distant metastases (group 3), and 92 patients with neither axillary nor distant metastatic disease (group 3). The average maximum SUV (obtained at a mean of 63 minutes after tracer administration) of the primary lesions in group 2 (7.7 plus or minus 6.2) was significantly higher than that in group 1 (4.8 plus or minus 3.9), followed by those in group 3 (2.9 plus or minus 2.7). The results of this study (**Figs. 5** and **6**) suggested that higher metabolic activity of the primary breast tumors as depicted by higher 18F-FDG accumulation can effectively

reflect the metastatic propensity of the tumor.[5] Hence, it can be perceived that higher breast tumor FDG accumulation in the primary lesion is commensurate with more disease burden at diagnosis (**Figs. 7–9**).

STUDIES INVESTIGATING FDG UPTAKE WITH TUMOR PROLIFERATION INDEX AND OTHER PARAMETERS

Two previous studies[6,7] have reported a significant correlation between [18F] FDG uptake in breast cancer by PET and proliferation index, percent Ki67 nuclear stain, in tumor tissue. In the study by Shimoda and colleagues,[7] a significant association was found between FDG accumulation and early and delayed-phase mitotic counts ($P = .0018$ and .0010, respectively), Ki67 positive cell percentage ($P = .0098$ and 0.0062, respectively), and nuclear

CASE 5

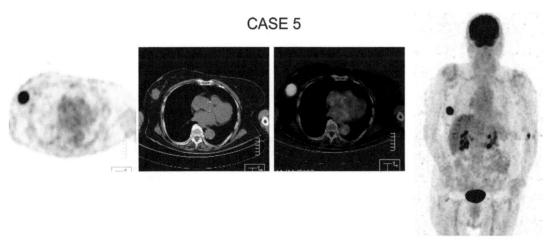

Fig. 4. Right breast invasive ductal and triple negative breast carcinoma (size 4.5 × 4 cm) and SUVmax: 14.

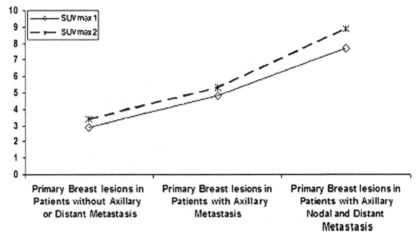

Fig. 5. Comparison of the SUVmax1 and the SUVmax2 values in the primary lesions in three different subgroups of patients with varying disease burden at diagnosis. (*Reprinted from* Basu S, Mavi A, Cermik T, et al. Implications of standardized uptake value measurements of the primary lesions in proven cases of breast carcinoma with different degree of disease burden at diagnosis: does 2-deoxy-2-[F-18]fluoro-D-glucose-positron emission tomography predict tumor biology? Mol Imaging Biol 2008;10(1):65; with permission.)

grade (P = .0232 and .0195, respectively). These investigators concluded that the biologic behavior of breast cancer is reflected in the variation of FDG uptake by the tumor.

Tchou and colleagues[8] examined the correlation of FDG uptake and percent Ki67 nuclear stain of tumor in a retrospective analysis in women with triple-negative breast cancer. As triple-negative cancers are more often poorly differentiated with a higher proliferation index, the authors

hypothesized that proliferation index of triple-negative breast cancer might correlate well with tumor glycolysis as measured by the uptake of FDG on PET. For this, the investigators calculated SUVmax in a group of 41 women, 22 with triple-negative and 19 with nontriple-negative breast cancer. FDG-PET imaging was significantly more sensitive in detecting triple-negative breast cancer than nontriple-negative breast cancer (95.5% vs 68.4%, P = .036). Triple-negative breast cancers

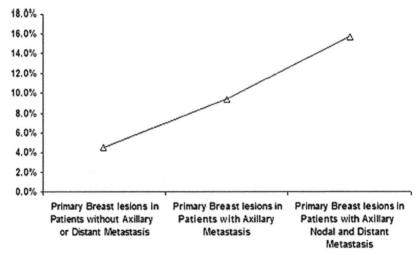

Fig. 6. Comparison of the %ΔSUVmax values in the primary lesions in three different subgroups of patients with varying disease burden at diagnosis. (*Reprinted from* Basu S, Mavi A, Cermik T, et al. Implications of standardized uptake value measurements of the primary lesions in proven cases of breast carcinoma with different degree of disease burden at diagnosis: does 2-deoxy-2-[F-18]fluoro-D-glucose-positron emission tomography predict tumor biology? Mol Imaging Biol 2008;10(1):66; with permission.)

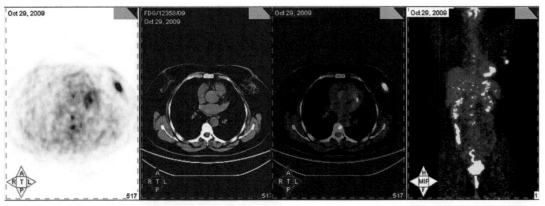

Fig. 7. A patient with left breast cancer with multiple left axillary lymph node metastases. Note the relatively intense FDG uptake despite being a small tumor (SUVmax: 5.4).

were noted to be poorly differentiated compared with nontriple-negative cancer ($P = .001$). FDG uptake correlated with proliferation index in women with triple-negative cancer. SUVmax correlated with percent Ki67 nuclear staining in the entire cohort (spearman correlation = 0.467, $P = .002$). Moreover, this significant correlation appeared to be driven primarily by a subset of women with triple-negative cancer (spearman correlation = 0.507, $P = .016$). This study[8] showed a significant correlation between proliferation index and FDG uptake, a biomarker that can be measured noninvasively and may facilitate clinical trials involving women with triple-negative breast cancer.

In their study, Bos and colleagues[9] compared FDG uptake in vivo with biomarkers expected to be involved in the underlying biologic mechanisms. Preoperative (18)FDG-PET scans were performed in 55 patients. The results demonstrated that FDG accumulation in the breast tumor is a function of microvasculature density for delivering nutrients ($P = .005$), GLUT1 for transportation of the tracer

into the cell ($P<.001$), hexokinase for entering the tracer into glycolysis ($P = .02$), number of viable cancerous cells per volume ($P = .009$), the proliferation rate ($P = .001$), the number of lymphocytes ($P = .03$), and the HIF-1a up-regulation of GLUT1. These characteristics, the authors concluded, would clarify why breast cancers vary in FDG uptake and elucidate the low uptake in lobular breast cancer. Another study by Burgman and colleagues[10] demonstrated that a hypoxia-induced increase in FDG accumulation in MCF-7 breast cancer cells is in part related to an increase in GLUT activity resulting from modification of the glucose transport proteins, whereas the modulation of hexokinase activity is probably not involved.

CORRELATION OF FDG UPTAKE AND OTHER PET PARAMETERS

In a study[11] to characterize and correlate the biologic response of locally advanced breast cancer (LABC) to chemotherapy using ^{15}O-water derived blood flow measurements and ^{18}F-FDG derived

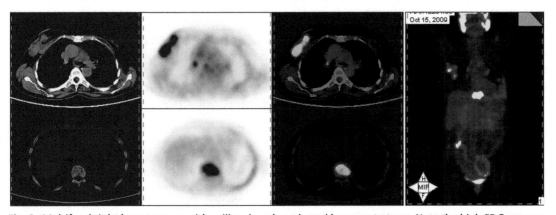

Fig. 8. Multifocal right breast cancer with axillary lymph node and bone metastases. Note the high FDG accumulation in the primary lesion (SUVmax: 6.3).

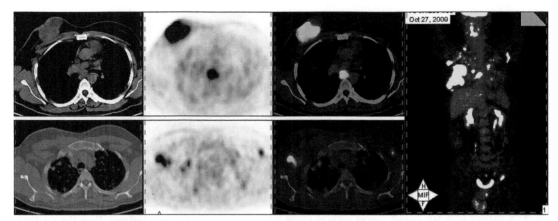

Fig. 9. A patient with right infiltrating duct carcinoma with multiple right axillary lymph nodes and bilateral pulmonary and bone metastases. The primary lesion shows very high FDG uptake (SUVmax: 10.9).

glucose metabolism rate parameters, 35 LABC patients were investigated using ^{15}O-water and ^{18}F-FDG PET before neoadjuvant chemotherapy and 2 months following initiation of therapy. Kinetic analysis for ^{15}O-water was performed using a single-tissue compartment model to calculate blood flow; a two-tissue compartment model was used to estimate ^{18}F-FDG rate parameters K_1, k_2, k_3, and the flux constant, K_i. Correlations and ratios between blood flow and ^{18}F-FDG rate parameters were calculated and compared with pathologic tumor response. Although blood flow and ^{18}F-FDG transport (K_1) were correlated before chemotherapy, there was relatively poor correlation between blood flow and the phosphorylation constant (k_3) or the overall ^{18}F-FDG flux (K_i). Blood flow and ^{18}F-FDG flux were more closely matched after chemotherapy, with changes in k_3 accounting for the increased correlation. These findings were consistent with a decline in both the K_i/flow and k_3/flow ratios with therapy. A low ratio of glucose metabolism (reflected by K_i) to glucose delivery (reflected by K_1 and blood flow) after therapy is associated with a favorable response. The authors concluded that the pattern of tumor glucose metabolism in LABC, as reflected by analysis of ^{18}F-FDG rate parameters, changes after therapy. This, according to these investigators, might indicate a change in tumor metabolic phenotype in response to therapy.

IN VITRO STUDIES IN BREAST CANCER CELL LINES

Several in vitro studies of human breast cancer cell lines have investigated the variation of GLUT receptors in various cells of different biologic characteristics. In one study involving different breast carcinoma cell lines, it was observed that cell surface GLUT1 expression was positively associated with cellular invasiveness, and GLUT2 and GLUT5 were inversely associated,[12] indirectly implying the possible role of FDG imaging in depicting invasiveness of breast carcinoma. In three different studies by Brown and colleagues,[13] the expression of GLUT1 and HK-II in animal tumor models of breast cancer and in women with untreated primary breast cancer[13–15] was examined. In the human studies, immunohistochemical staining showed that 61% of tumors were positive for GLUT1, and 79% of tumors were positive for HK-II.[13] Cells that expressed HK-II did not always express GLUT1 and vise versa. A point of note is that FDG uptake appeared to be associated with increased GLUT1 expression (P = .02) but not with HK-II expression (P = .6).[13] Recently, GLUT12, a novel GLUT protein, located intracellularly and at the cell surface,[16] has been implicated in determining breast cancer biology. Trafficking of intracellular GLUT12 to the plasma membrane may contribute to the enhanced glucose accumulation in breast cancer. Macheda and colleagues[17] observed that estradiol and epidermal growth factor increase GLUT12 protein levels in cultured breast cancer cells,[17] implying that GLUT12 may be a novel targeting agent for detecting and treating breast cancer.

FUTURE DIRECTIONS

The potential of metabolic and molecular imaging with PET in elucidating tumor biology in breast carcinoma appears substantial at this time. This adds to the initial endeavors[18,19] that primarily were directed at the use of FDG-PET in detection and staging. PET led by FDG imaging is likely to be at the forefront of cancer imaging in the future. The relation between FDG uptake with that of novel PET tracers may provide better insight into the tumor pathophysiology and may aid in evolving and adapting newer therapeutics in the clinical research and practice of breast cancer treatment.

REFERENCES

1. Buck A, Schirrmeister H, Kuhn T, et al. FDG uptake in breast cancer: correlation with biological and clinical prognostic parameters. Eur J Nucl Med Mol Imaging 2002;29:1317–23.

2. Crippa F, Seregni E, Agresti R, et al. Association between [18F]-fluorodeoxyglucose uptake and postoperative histopathology, hormone receptor status, thymidine labeling index, and p53 in primary breast cancer: a preliminary observation. Eur J Nucl Med 1998;25:1429–34.

3. Basu S, Chen W, Tchou J, et al. Comparison of triple-negative and estrogen receptor-positive/progesterone receptor-positive/HER2-negative breast carcinoma using quantitative fluorine-18 fluorodeoxyglucose/positron emission tomography imaging parameters: a potentially useful method for disease characterization. Cancer 2008;112(5):995–1000.

4. Mavi A, Cermik TF, Urhan M, et al. The effects of estrogen, progesterone, and C-erbB-2 receptor states on 18F-FDG uptake of primary breast cancer lesions. J Nucl Med 2007;48(8):1266–72.

5. Basu S, Mavi A, Cermik T, et al. Implications of standardized uptake value measurements of the primary lesions in proven cases of breast carcinoma with different degree of disease burden at diagnosis: does 2-deoxy-2-[F-18]fluoro-D-glucose-positron emission tomography predict tumor biology? Mol Imaging Biol 2008;10(1):62–6.

6. Avril N, Rose CA, Schelling M, et al. Breast imaging with positron emission tomography and fluorine-18 fluorodeoxyglucose: use and limitations. J Clin Oncol 2000;18(20):3495–502.

7. Shimoda W, Hayashi M, Murakami K, et al. The relationship between FDG uptake in PET scans and biological behavior in breast cancer. Breast Cancer 2007;14(3):260–8.

8. Tchou J, Sonnad S, Bergey MR, et al. Degree of tumor FDG uptake correlates with proliferation index in triple-negative breast cancer. Mol Imaging Biol 2009. [Epub ahead of print].

9. Bos R, van Der Hoeven JJ, van Der Wall E, et al. Biologic correlates of 18fluorodeoxyglucose uptake in human breast cancer measured by positron emission tomography. J Clin Oncol 2002;20:379–87.

10. Burgman P, O'Donoghue JA, Humm JL, et al. Hypoxia-induced increase in FDG uptake in MCF7 cells. J Nucl Med 2001;42:170–5.

11. Tseng J, Dunnwald LK, Schubert EK, et al. 18F-FDG kinetics in locally advanced breast cancer: correlation with tumor blood flow and changes in response to neoadjuvant chemotherapy. J Nucl Med 2004; 45(11):1829–37.

12. Grover-McKay M, Walsh SA, Seftor EA, et al. Role for glucose transporter 1protein in human breast cancer. Pathol Oncol Res 1998;4:115–20.

13. Brown RS, Goodman TM, Zasadny KR, et al. Expression of hexokinase II and glut-1 in untreated human breast cancer. Nucl Med Biol 2002;29:443–53.

14. Brown RS, Leung JY, Fisher SJ, et al. Intratumoral distribution of tritiated-FDG in breast carcinoma: correlation between glut-1 expression and FDG uptake. J Nucl Med 1996;37:1042–7.

15. Brown RS, Wahl RL. Overexpression of glut-1 glucose transporter in human breast cancer: an immunohistochemical study. Cancer 1993;72:2979–85.

16. Rogers S, Macheda ML, Docherty SE, et al. Identification of a novel glucose transporter-like protein-glut-12. Am J Physiol Endocrinol Metab 2002;282: E733–8.

17. Macheda ML, Rogers S, Bets JD. Molecular and cellular regulation of glucose transport (GLUT) proteins in cancer. J Cell Physiol 2005;202:654–62.

18. Kumar R, Loving VA, Chauhan A, et al. Potential of dual-time-point imaging to improve breast cancer diagnosis with (18)F-FDG PET. J Nucl Med 2005; 46(11):1819–24.

19. Mavi A, Urhan M, Yu JQ, et al. Dual time point 18F-FDG PET imaging detects breast cancer with high sensitivity and correlates well with histologic subtypes. J Nucl Med 2006;47(9):1440–6.

Role of [F-18] 2-Deoxy-2-Fluoro-D-Glucose PET and PET/CT in Staging and Follow-Up of Breast Cancer

Tevfik Fikret Çermik, MD[a], Ayşe Mavi, MD[b],
Abass Alavi, MD, MD (Hon), PhD (Hon), Dsc (Hon)[c,*]

KEYWORDS

- FDG-PET or PET/CT • Breast cancer
- Staging • Restaging • Recurrent • Metastasis

Breast cancer is the most common malignancy that affects women in most Western countries, accounting for approximately 25% of all cancers in female patients, and is also the second leading cause of cancer-related death in this population. Although the incidence of breast cancer has increased by 10% to 15% over the last 30 years, the overall mortality rate has remained relatively stable. The main prognostic factors in patients with breast cancer are tumor size, histologic grade, estrogen receptor state, axillary lymph node state, and the presence or absence of distant metastasis. Overall, 5-year survival rates are approximately 75%, with a range of 92% for stage I to 15% for stage IV disease.[1] For this reason, accurate staging of breast cancer at the time of the initial diagnosis and in the follow-up period has a major impact on the choice of therapeutic modalities that are selected for optimal management of these patients. This article focuses on the role of [18]F 2-deoxy-2-fluoro-D-glucose (FDG)-PET and PET combined with computed tomography (PET/CT) in the preoperative staging of primary breast cancer, and assessment of recurrent and metastatic disease in the follow-up period.

DIAGNOSIS OF PRIMARY TUMORS

Most primary breast tumors are initially detected either by self-examination or routine breast examinations to investigate a suspicious mass. Unfortunately, most of the tumors are smaller than 1 cm in diameter and are usually not palpable. Because of the difference in size and density of the breasts, physical examination of the breast generally does not permit an accurate differentiation between a malignant and nonmalignant mass.[2]

Conventional or digital mammography has been shown to be a sensitive method for breast cancer screening, with the exception of some specific situations such as dense breast and the presence of extensive scarring from prior biopsies. Mammography allows the detection of breast masses earlier than physical examination. However, both malignant and benign breast lesions often display a similar diagnostic appearance,

[a] Clinic of Nuclear Medicine, Istanbul Education and Research Hospital, Samatya, Fatih, Istanbul 34310, Turkey
[b] Department of Nuclear Medicine, Yeditepe University Hospital, Devlet Yolu Ankara Caddesi No: 102/104, Kozyatagi, Istanbul 34752, Turkey
[c] Division of Nuclear Medicine, Department of Radiology, Hospital of the University of Pennsylvania, 3400 Spruce Street, 110 Donner Building, Philadelphia, PA 19104, USA
* Corresponding author.
E-mail address: alavi@rad.upenn.edu (A. Alavi).

PET Clin 4 (2009) 391–404
doi:10.1016/j.cpet.2009.11.001
1556-8598/09/$ – see front matter © 2009 Published by Elsevier Inc.

and this is a major diagnostic challenge for mammography.[3] Positive predictive value (PPV) of mammography is 10% to 35% for nonpalpable breast cancers, and the frequency of positive biopsy findings after abnormal mammography can be as low as 10%.[3–5]

The first FDG imaging with PET was reported in 1989 by Kubota and colleagues[6] in a patient with breast cancer with local recurrence. Until today, FDG-PET has been shown to be a useful technique for breast cancer management by various investigators. Previous studies about breast cancer using FDG-PET were limited by the small number of patients and high prevalence of malignant tumors. Wahl and colleagues[7] first reported increased FDG uptake in 10 patients with breast cancer who had locally advanced and metastatic disease. This first study of Wahl and colleagues succeeded in detecting primary lesions of breast cancer. However, the study was limited to large primary lesions and could not adequately detect smaller lesions in the breast. In a prospective study with a larger population, Adler and colleagues[8] investigated 28 patients with primary breast cancer and 7 patients with benign lesions and correctly identified 27 of 28 malignant tumors, with a sensitivity of 96% and a specificity of 100%. In this study, there was a significant correlation between the nuclear grade of the tumors and the uptake value of FDG. Dehdashti and colleagues[9] assessed 24 malignant and 8 benign breast lesions using FDG-PET, and they found standard uptake value (SUV) of FDG to be much higher in breast cancer than in the nonmalignant lesions (4.5 ± 2.8 vs 1.0 ± 0.4). Although previously mentioned studies have reported the utility of FDG-PET imaging in assessing patients with primary breast cancer, 2 studies stood out for their large number of patient series.[10,11] The study by Avril and colleagues,[10] which included 144 cases, is the one that has the largest number of patients with breast cancer examined by FDG-PET. In this study, images were evaluated by 2 different reading methods. The sensitivity of FDG-PET by the "sensitive image reading method" was determined as follows: 42% for Tis, 25% for T1a to T1b, 84% for T1c, 92% for T2, and 100% for T3. The overall sensitivity, specificity, PPV, negative predictive value (NPV), and accuracy in this study were 80%, 75%, 89%, 61%, and 79%, respectively. Sixty-five percent of invasive lobular cancers and 24% of invasive ductal cancers were FDG-PET negative in this study, and there was a clear relationship between tumor size and lesion detectability. The corresponding values for the second series, which consisted of 117 patients, were 93%, 75%, 92%, 78%, and 89%,

respectively, but no values were given for each T stage.[11] Cermik and colleagues[12] reported in their prospective study that increased maximum SUV (SUVmax) is associated with higher TNM stage of the disease. In this study, the differences between SUVmax in TNM stage II, III, and IV are independent of tumor sizes, and significant differences are noted in SUVmax of lesions according to pathologic T stages. The sensitivity rates for FDG-PET in this study were determined as follows: 72% for Tis, 53% for T1mic and T1a, 63% for T1b, 80% for T1c, and 92% for T2 and T3.

Multifocal or multicentric breast cancer is an important entity of breast cancer, and was not reported adequately by using PET (**Fig. 1**). Schirrmeister and colleagues[11] reported that FDG-PET was 2 times more sensitive in the diagnoses of multifocal lesions than a combination of mammography and ultrasonography. However, Avril and colleagues[10] reported that only 50% of multifocal or multicentric breast cancers were identified by FDG-PET. FDG-PET has a lower sensitivity compared with MRI because of limited spatial resolution. MRI can provide detailed information about the size and the local extension of primary breast cancer and evaluate multifocal or multicentric tumors.[13] Uematsu and colleagues[14] reported that MRI was significantly more accurate than FDG-PET in the assessment of tumor extent of breast cancers. In their study, the accuracy of FDG-PET (43%) was significantly lower than that of MRI (91%) when assessing the local extent of primary tumors. Similarly, MRI has been reported to be the most accurate breast imaging modality compared with multidetector CT, ultrasonography, and mammography for the detection of tumor extension of breast cancer.[15]

The detection rate of breast cancer by FDG-PET has been reported to be lower when the tumor diameter is less than 1 cm owing to a partial volume effect; this is especially true for well-differentiated tumors (tubular carcinomas, lobular carcinomas, and carcinoma in situ).[16,17] Single-time-point PET performed 1 hour after the injection of FDG could be a suboptimal method for assessment of suspected breast cancer. It is well known that the uptake of FDG increases over several hours in most malignancies, and therefore, it would be more accurate to obtain an additional delayed image (dual time-point imaging) 90 to 120 minutes after FDG injection.[18,19] It has been shown that most of the breast cancers demonstrate a gradual increase in SUV with time after FDG injection, like most other cancers.[20,21] Mavi and colleagues performed dual time-point imaging of 152 patients with breast cancers. The SUVmax of FDG was measured at both time points. The

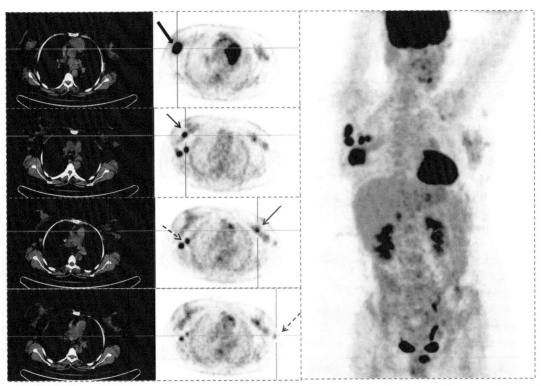

Fig. 1. FDG-PET/CT transaxial slices and anterior maximum intensity projection of a 41-year-old woman diagnosed with breast cancer and referred for initial staging demonstrated right multicentric (*thick and thin black arrows*) and left single (*red arrow*) primary malignant mass and bilateral axillary lymph node metastases (*dashed arrows*).

percent change in SUVmax (Δ%SUVmax) between time points 1 (SUVmax1) and 2 (SUVmax2) was calculated for invasive and noninvasive malignant lesions and contralateral normal breast tissues. The mean ± SD of the SUVmax1, the SUVmax2, and the Δ%SUVmax were 3.9 ± 3.7, 4.3 ± 4.0, and 8.3% ± 11.5% for invasive; 2.0 ± 0.6, 2.1 ± 0.6, and 3.4% ± 13.0% for noninvasive; and 1.2 ± 0.3, 1.1 ± 0.2, and −10.0% ± 10.8% for the contralateral normal breast groups, respectively. SUVmax increased over time in both invasive and noninvasive tumors, whereas the physiologic uptake of normal breast tissue significantly decreased over time. Visual assessment revealed that the sensitivity of dual time-point imaging was 90% for invasive cancer larger than 10 mm, 83% for tumors that are 4 to 10 mm, and 77% for noninvasive breast cancers. The investigators suggested that dual time-point imaging may improve the sensitivity and accuracy of FDG-PET in assessing patients with primary breast cancers.[22]

Similar to other 3D imaging techniques, PET scans study patients in the supine position. However, this position can provide motion-related artifacts for breast tissue caused by patients' respiration during long study periods of PET imaging. Yutani and colleagues[23] recommended prone position in PET imaging for detection of breast cancer. Kaida and colleagues[24] performed supine whole body and prone breast FDG-PET imaging in 118 patients with breast cancers. These investigators reported that 10 of 114 malignant breast lesions (9%) were detected only in prone breast images. The sensitivity and accuracy of prone breast PET were 95% and 93%, respectively, and statistically significant difference was found between the sensitivity and accuracy of prone breast PET images and those of whole body PET images. In addition, prone position may separate deep breast lesions from the myocardium, liver, and chest wall muscles by decreasing scatter from FDG uptake in these organs compared with supine position.

Integrated PET/CT, which combines anatomic and metabolic imaging information, has been shown to further improve diagnostic accuracy and clinical management of patients through accurate localization of functional data on high-resolution anatomic CT images.[25,26] Although PET/CT devices have improved technologically in time, FDG-PET/CT still does not have adequate

Table 1
FDG-PET and PET/CT results for detection of axillary lymph node metastases

Investigators and Year of Study (ref.)	No. of Patients	Sensitivity (%)	Specificity (%)
Utech et al, 1996[32]	124	100	75
Avril et al, 1996[33]	51	79	96
Adler et al, 1997[34]	52	95	66
Smith et al, 1998[35]	50	90	97
Crippa et al, 1998[36]	72	85	91
Rostom et al, 1999[37]	74	86	100
Schirrmeister et al, 2001[11]	85	79	92
Greco et al, 2001[38]	167	94	86
van der Hoeven et al, 2002[39]	70	25	97
Wahl et al, 2004[40]	308	61	83
Lovrics et al, 2004[41]	98	40	97
Chung et al, 2006[42]	51	64	89
Gil-Rendo et al, 2006[43]	275	84	98
Cermik et al, 2007[12]	271	56	89
Heusner et al, 2009[44]	61	58	92
Kim et al, 2009[45]	137	77	100

performance for initial diagnosis of patients with T1 breast tumors. A recently published article by Imbriaco and colleagues[27] evaluated 55 breast lesions. The patients underwent dual time-point FDG-PET/CT in the prone position and breast MRI. In their study, MRI showed an overall accuracy of 95%, with sensitivity and specificity of 98% and 80%, respectively. However, dual time-point PET/CT had an accuracy of 84% for lesions with an SUVmax higher than 2.5 or positive Δ%SUVmax, with sensitivity and specificity of 80% and 100%. The results of several FGD-PET and PET/CT studies showed that currently, the role of FDG-PET or PET/CT is not efficient in detection of primary lesions.

AXILLARY LYMPH NODE STAGING

The most common sites of regional metastasis of breast cancer are the axillary lymph nodes. Axillary lymph node status in the newly diagnosed breast cancer is the most powerful indicator of prognosis and the most important factor in determining the treatment modality for an individual. The 10-year survival rate in patients with axillary lymph node metastases depends on the number of involved nodes and ranges from 30% to 70% compared with 90% in those without involvement.[28,29] Clinical examination of axilla is generally unreliable for staging, and currently there is a need for an

accurate structural or functional imaging technique that can detect axillary lymph node metastasis with high reliability. Therefore, standardized axillary lymph node dissection (ALND) continues to be the best procedure for examining the lymph nodes. However, ALND can be the cause of a significant morbidity such as lymphedema, pain, or restriction of shoulder and arm movements.[30] Up to 70% of patients who have stage T1 and T2 tumors have negative axillary nodes.[31]

Several studies have been reported for the use of FDG-PET in detecting axillary lymph node involvement over the past 2 decades. Most of these research studies demonstrated that the sensitivity ranges from 25% to 100% and the specificity from 66% to 100% for the detection of axillary involvement in patients with breast cancer by FDG-PET (**Table 1**).[11,32–40,43] The leading cause of such significant variations among the studies is the difference in the selection criteria for study populations enrolled. It is plausible to hypothesize that the sensitivity of FDG-PET for the detection of axillary lymph node involvement in study groups increases with higher stages of disease. By considering the studies with large numbers of patients, the axillary metastasis rate was calculated to be between 35% and 44% as confirmed by the histologic evaluation.[11,36,38,40,41] Greco and colleagues[38] studied 167 consecutive patients with breast cancer, and in their study axillary metastasis rate was found to be 43%, which was also verified by histologic evaluation in their study group. In this study the sensitivity, specificity, and accuracy rates of FDG-PET for the primary tumor were determined to be 94%, 86%, and 90%, respectively. There were only 4 false negative PET scans in 72 patients and all of them had micrometastasis. However, in their study, enrolled patients had a higher T stage, and axillary staging was conducted according to clinical results. Subsequently, 3 remarkable studies were performed concerning the role of FDG-PET in detecting axillary lymph node involvement. The first of these studies was conducted by Wahl and colleagues.[40] The study included 360 patients and reported an axillary metastasis detection rate of 35% after histologic analysis. In this study, the data from 3 different centers were evaluated separately, and the overall sensitivity, specificity, PPV, and NPV were found to be 61%, 80%, 62%, and 79%, respectively. The sensitivity and PPV were found to be remarkably low compared with the studies published before 2000, and the investigators concluded that FDG-PET is not recommended routinely for axillary staging in patients with breast cancer. Further studies using FDG-PET confirm the relatively low sensitivity for axillary nodal metastases in early-stage breast cancer.[39,41,42] Another study that has a large group of patients was performed by Gil-Rendo and colleagues.[43] In this study, relatively higher sensitivity rates for axillary state were detected in comparison with the other studies mentioned here. The study included 2 groups. In the first group of 150 women who had preoperative FDG-PET and ALND, the sensitivity and specificity of FDG-PET for detecting axillary state were 90% and 99%, respectively. Adjuvant intraoperative sentinel node biopsy (SNB) was performed in the second group of 125 patients, who had negative axillary PET images. The sensitivity and specificity of PET for detecting axillary involvement were 81% in N1, 92% in N2, and 87% in N3 stages, and overall sensitivity and specificity were 79% and 98%, respectively. In the third study, Cermik and colleagues[12] reported data obtained from 271 patients with newly diagnosed breast cancer who had SNB or ALND after FDG-PET scans. This study had one of the largest groups of patients enrolled at a single site, and obtained axillary metastatic rates that are similar to those of the other studies mentioned here. Axillary involvement rate was found to be 34% after histologic analysis. In their study, the sensitivity for detecting axillary lymph node metastasis was found to be 41% in pN1, 67% in pN2, and 100% in pN3, and

specificity was 89% for stage pN0. The investigators suggested that the main reason for low sensitivity in low stages is the relatively high rate of micrometastasis. Only 2 axillary involvements were positive on FDG-PET scans, whereas micrometastasis was revealed in 18 patients in their study group. Heusner and colleagues[44] recently found similar lower sensitivity in the diagnosis of axillary involvement in 61 patients using PET/CT, and the sensitivity, specificity, PPV, and NPV rates were 58%, 92%, 82%, and 77%, respectively. These studies clearly indicate the limitation of FDG-PET and PET/CT for axillary staging because of lower sensitivity in N1 to N2 and T1 stages.

At present, SNB has been described as the most accurate method for assessing axillary nodal status to determine whether to perform ALND.[41] The morbidity of SNB is less than that of ALND, and the procedure may improve staging of axilla.[46] In recent years, there has been a general consensus on the application of SNB in unifocal primary tumors with a maximum size of 2 to 3 cm and without clinical suspicion of axillary lymph node metastases.[44] However, the false negative rate of SNB is an important problem in the management of axilla. The main cause of false negatives in SNB is skip metastasis, which is found in 4% to 10% of the patients with axillary metastasis.[47,48] For this reason, axillary involvement on the FDG-PET or PET/CT can help in avoiding SNB. In a recent series,[45] either ALND or SNB was performed on 137 biopsy-proven patients with breast cancer, and the results were compared with the PET/CT axillary lymph node status. Twenty-seven patients who had positive PET/CT underwent complete ALND as a primary procedure, and 110 patients with negative PET/CT underwent SNB and additional non-SNB. False negative scans were found in 8 patients. Overall sensitivity, specificity, and PPV of FDG-PET/CT in predicting axillary metastasis were 77%, 100%, and 100%, respectively. The results of all these FDG-PET and PET/CT studies showed that these diagnostic methods still cannot replace SNB in the near future in the management of breast cancers.

INTERNAL MAMMARY, EXTRA-AXILLARY REGIONAL, AND INTRATHORACIC LYMPH NODE STATUS

Conventional diagnostic techniques are not considered optimal in detecting metastasis of internal mammary nodes. In addition, the tissue sampling of these lymph nodes is not routinely performed at the surgery, and therefore the importance of internal mammary lymph chain involvement still cannot be evaluated properly. Metastasis of the internal mammary nodes in the absence of axillary nodal involvement is approximately 4% to 6%,[49,50] and is frequently seen in advanced stages of the disease or is associated with distant metastases.[51,52]

Eubank and colleagues reported that mediastinal and internal mammary lymph node metastases were seen twice as often as FDG-PET compared with CT in 73 patients with recurrent or metastatic breast cancer. FDG-PET has shown that 40% of the patients had intrathoracic lymph node metastases, and only 23% of these patients had enlarged nodes in CT.[53] The sensitivity and specificity of FDG-PET for nodal disease were 85% and 90%, whereas the same rates for CT were 54% and 85%, respectively, after the histologic analysis or follow-up results. In the locoregional advanced breast cancer patients group, internal mammary involvement was detected in only 7 of 28 women by FDG-PET. No pathologic findings were noted in CT of the thorax.[51] In Cermik and colleagues' study,[12] 13 (6%) patients showed extra-axillary locoregional lymph node involvement on FDG-PET scan, whereas 7 of 13 patients had ipsilateral internal mammary lymph node metastases. However, CT was negative in these 7 patients. In the study group, 6 patients had ipsilateral infra- or supraclavicular and 8 patients had intrathoracic or abdominal lymph node metastases. Heusner and colleagues[54] reported recently that 3 of 40 patients having extra-axillary lymph node metastases were detected only by PET/CT. Overall, several of the reported studies have definitely demonstrated that FDG-PET is superior to conventional diagnostic techniques, such as CT, in the detection of locoregional lymph node metastases, particularly to the internal mammary regions, and intrathoracic lymph node involvement. FDG-PET and PET/CT may be helpful in the selection of patients who would benefit from radiation therapy on the internal mammary lymph chain.

DISTANT METASTATIC DISEASE

The presence of distant metastases is an important prognostic factor in patients with newly diagnosed breast cancer. Also, metastatic state of the disease affects therapeutic options. Current methods for the detection of distant metastasis at the time of initial diagnosis of breast cancer include chest radiography, liver ultrasonography (US), bone scan, CT, and MRI. Distant metastases in several studies have been diagnosed by using chest radiography, liver US, and bone scan. In these studies, total metastasis detection rate

was 3.4% to 3.9%, and it was less than 1% for lung and liver metastasis in newly diagnosed patients with breast cancer.[55–57] It is well known that the bone is the most common site of distant metastasis, and metastases to the bone are diagnosed in 30% to 85% of patients with advanced breast cancer.[58]

The role of FDG-PET and PET/CT in detecting distant metastases and the comparison of results with conventional imaging methods in breast cancer have been well defined in the literature in last decade. In a study by Schirrmeister and colleagues,[11] which consisted of 93 patients, distant metastases were revealed in 6 patients by FDG-PET. In another study that included 84 newly diagnosed patients with breast cancer, distant metastases were detected in 4 cases on the FDG-PET and confirmed radiologically.[59] In a study by Cermik and colleagues[12] involving 246 patients with invasive breast cancer, bone and bone marrow were the most common distant metastatic sites. Skeletal metastasis was found in 8 (3.2%) patients, and metastatic involvement of the lung and liver in 4 (1.6%) and 2 (0.8%), respectively, on FDG-PET scan. The results of these 3 studies using FDG-PET showed distant metastatic lesions in the bone, lung, and liver similar to conventional imaging techniques. However, FDG-PET seems to be a limited contributor in the detection of distant metastatic lesions at the time of primary diagnosis of patients with breast cancer, especially in low stages.

Fuster and colleagues[60] studied 60 consecutive patients with large (>3 cm) primary breast cancer. FDG-PET/CT diagnosed 6 bone, 2 lung, and 2 liver metastases in 8 (13%) patients, whereas there were no findings by conventional workup in these patients. The sensitivity and specificity of PET/CT in detecting distant metastasis were 100% and 98%, respectively, whereas conventional workup (chest CT, liver US and bone scan) sensitivity and specificity were found to be 60% and 83%, respectively. In another recently published study of 69 patients with locally advanced breast cancer, it was reported that 19 patients had lung, liver, or bone metastases.[61] Conventional imaging methods detected distant metastases in 8 of these 19 patients (42%), whereas FDG-PET detected metastatic disease in 18 patients (95%). The liver and bone metastases were missed by FDG-PET in only 1 patient in this study group.

Inflammatory breast cancer is the most aggressive type of breast cancer, characterized by high rates of distant metastasis in the primary diagnosis and follow-up period. It also has a higher locoregional recurrence rate compared with other types of breast malignancies. In a retrospective study of 41 patients with initial-staging inflammatory breast cancer, FDG-PET/CT demonstrated distant metastasis in 20 patients; only 13 of them had positive metastatic findings on conventional imaging methods.[62]

Based on these findings, FDG-PET and PET/CT seem to detect much more distant metastatic lesions compared with conventional imaging methods in locally advanced and inflammatory breast cancers (**Figs. 2 and 3**). However, current PET devices have a lower sensitivity in assessing lung nodules smaller than 1 cm, because of partial volume effect and respiratory motion. In such cases, CT images on PET/CT can be very helpful in the assessment of small nodules arising from metastatic pulmonary disease.

Bone marrow and osteolytic bone metastases have been shown to be more common than osteosclerotic (osteoblastic) bone metastasis in newly diagnosed breast cancer.[63–66] Cook and colleagues[63] reported that FDG-PET was more sensitive than bone scan in detecting osseous lesions, and PET seems to be superior to bone scan for assessment of bone metastasis in newly diagnosed patients with breast cancer. Some other reports have shown no difference between the sensitivity of these 2 methods. However, the specificity and overall accuracy of FDG-PET have been noted to be higher in some reports.[67,68] In contrast, there was no significant difference in the sensitivity and the specificity of FDG-PET and bone scan results in patients during the

follow-up period.[69–71] These studies showed that FDG-PET tends to be superior to bone scan in the detection of osteolytic lesions, but inferior in the detection of osteoblastic lesions. Similarly, Nakai and colleagues[72] demonstrated that FDG-PET had sensitivities of 56%, 100%, and 95%, respectively, for the detection of osteoblastic, osteolytic, and mixed lesions, whereas bone scan had sensitivities of 100%, 70%, and 84%, respectively. While bone scan reveals the osteoblastic reaction of the bone tissue against metastasis to the red marrow, FDG-PET imaging visualizes enhanced glucolytic metabolism of the viable tumor cell in the skeleton. The malignant cell content of osteoblastic metastases is lower than that of osteolytic lesions. This concept is supported by the fact that patients with osteoblastic metastases are known to survive longer compared with those with osteolytic metastases.[73]

RECURRENT DISEASE

Locoregional recurrence after the initial diagnosis and treatment of breast cancer occurs in 7% to 30% of patients.[74] The recurrence most frequently involves the breast and the chest wall. Axillary and supraclavicular nodes are also frequently involved. Clinical detection and conventional imaging of locoregional recurrence are difficult because the findings of locoregional recurrence cannot be reliably distinguished from posttherapeutic changes. In current clinical practice, patients with breast

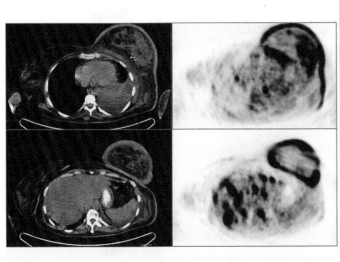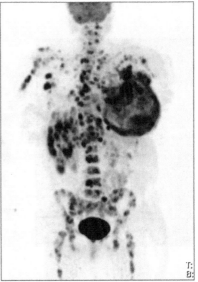

Fig. 2. A 44-year-old woman with invasive ductal carcinoma underwent FDG-PET/CT for initial staging. Transaxial slices and anterior MIP showed primary tumor and skin invasion of the left breast. Images also demonstrated multiple liver and skeletal metastases.

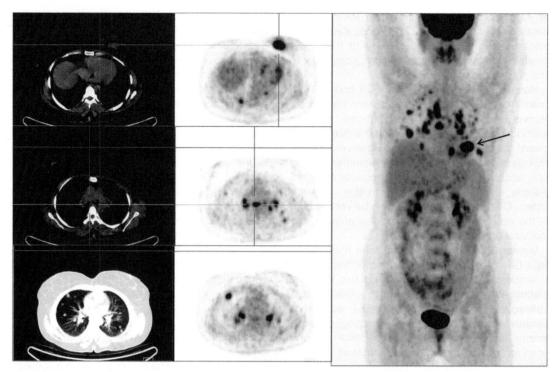

Fig. 3. FDG-PET/CT of a 38-year-old woman with invasive ductal carcinoma who came for initial staging. Transaxial PET/CT images and MIP demonstrated primary lesion of the left breast, multiple lung and mediastinal lymph node metastases. There were no clinical or PET/CT findings of the axillary lymph node metastasis in this patient.

cancer regularly undergo mammography every 1 to 2 years to check for local recurrence or contralateral second cancer. The most common distant metastatic site is bone, followed by lung and liver, in the follow-up period. The imaging studies such as chest radiography, liver ultrasonography, chest and abdominal CT and bone scans, breast MRI, and FDG-PET are used for the diagnosis of distant

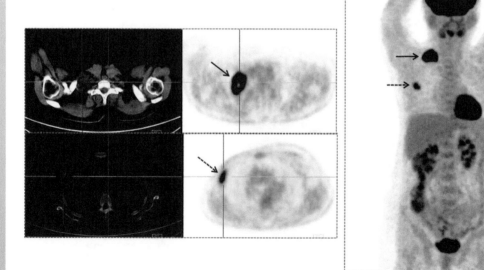

Fig. 4. A 45-year-old patient underwent PET/CT for restaging. There was a suspicion of having metastatic disease because of palpable supraclavicular masses. Transaxial slices demonstrated right chest wall recurrent lesion (*dashed arrow*) and metastatic supraclavicular lymph nodes (*black arrow*).

metastasis, but none of them are recommended for breast cancer surveillance in current clinical practice.[75]

Conventional imaging techniques are limited in differentiating posttherapeutic changes from tumor recurrence, and it can be difficult to characterize and differentiate small foci of early metastatic disease from benign lesions. However, FDG-PET or PET/CT seems to be the most useful method compared with conventional imaging studies for restaging those patients with suspected recurrence in breast cancer. This approach is especially valuable in the assessment of regions that have been previously treated by surgery and radiation.[76] Moon and colleagues[69] investigated 57 patients with breast cancer having clinical or radiological suspicion of recurrent or metastatic disease after treatment by using FDG-PET. In this study the reported sensitivity, specificity, PPV, and NPV for the detection of recurrent

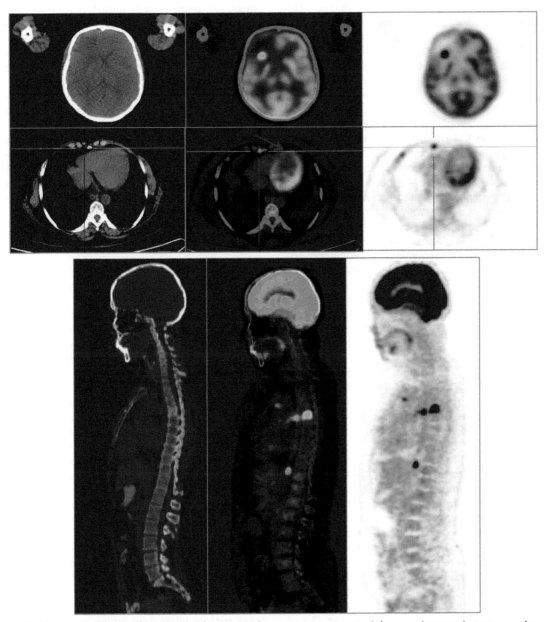

Fig. 5. PET/CT of a 46-year-old patient with suspected recurrence or metastasis because increase in tumor markers was shown. Transaxial cranial slice showed a metastatic brain lesion (*black arrow*), and thoracic slice demonstrated chest wall (*red arrow*) and internal mammary lymph node metastases (*target*). Sagittal slice also showed fifth thoracic vertebral metastasis.

disease were 93%, 79%, 82%, and 92%, respectively. In a retrospective analysis of 62 patients in the follow-up period, Gallowitsch and colleagues[77] compared FGD-PET with conventional imaging including mammography, US, CT and MRI, and bone scans. Sensitivity, specificity, PPV, and NPV of FDG-PET for detecting local recurrence or distant metastases were 97%, 82%, 87%, and 96%, respectively. For comparison, the corresponding values for conventional imaging methods were 84%, 60%, 75%, and 73%, respectively. Wolfort and colleagues[78] studied 171 patients with stage I and II breast cancers, and 23 patients met their criteria of clinical suspicion of recurrence (an abnormal mammography, a palpable mass at the surgical site, or symptoms of local or distant metastasis). Overall sensitivity, specificity, PPV, and NPV of FDG-PET were 81%, 100%, 100%, and 50%, respectively.

Carcinoembryonic antigen (CEA) and cancer antigen 15-3 (CA 15-3) are the most frequently used tumor markers for the detection of asymptomatic recurrences of breast cancer in postsurgical follow-up.[79] However, these tumor markers have a low specificity, and increased levels do not always correlate with recurrence. Liu and colleagues[80] studied 28 patients with recurrent breast cancer who had asymptomatic tumor marker increase but negative or equivocal conventional imaging results. These investigators reported that FDG-PET accurately detected 25 of 28 patients with recurrence, and the sensitivity and accuracy of PET in this group were 96% and 90%, respectively. Suarez and colleagues[81] performed FDG-PET studies in 38 patients with increased CEA or CA 15-3 and no findings of recurrence on conventional imaging. Tumor marker-guided PET images correctly identified 24 of 26 recurrent and 9 of 12 nonrecurrent patients and the sensitivity, specificity, PPV, and NPV were 92%, 75%, 89%, and 82%, respectively.

According to the literature, the PET/CT scanner with fusion images provides more precise anatomic definition for uptake localization, which can increase sensitivity and specificity.[82–84] At present, there are not enough published reports regarding the role of FDG-PET/CT systems in the assessment of recurrent diseases in patients with breast cancer. A recent article by Piperkova and colleagues[85] compared FDG-PET/CT with contrast-enhanced CT in assessment of the locoregional or distant metastatic lesions in 70 studies of 49 patients with breast cancer. Out of a total of 257 lesions, 210 were concordant between the 2 methods. There were 47 discordant lesions found, which were verified by either biopsy

or follow-up. While PET/CT identified 25 lesions correctly and 2 incorrectly, CT identified 2 lesions correctly and 18 lesions incorrectly of these 47 discordant lesions. The sensitivity, specificity, PPV, and NPV for PET/CT were 98%, 93%, 99%, and 85% and for CT 88%, 42%, 92%, and 32%, respectively. Tatsumi and colleagues[86] studied 61 patients with suspected recurrence or for follow-up assessment. In their study, it was reported that PET/CT demonstrated a significantly better accuracy than CT. PET/CT accurately staged 52 patients with malignancies, whereas CT accurately evaluated 47. Similarly, Radan and colleagues[87] reported that in patients with suspected recurrences because of elevated tumor markers, FDG-PET/CT had a better performance than CT for the diagnosis of tumor recurrences. In this study, PET/CT had a higher sensitivity (85% vs 70%), specificity (76% vs 47%), and accuracy (81% vs 59%) compared with contrast-enhanced CT. The results of these 3 studies demonstrated that PET/CT has a more reliable role than CT alone and therefore, PET/CT had some impact on the management of breast cancers during the follow-up period (**Figs. 4** and **5**).

SUMMARY

The precise role of PET/CT continues to evolve even 20 years after the first study using FDG-PET for the assessment of breast cancers. PET and PET/CT devices still do not achieve adequate accuracy for the diagnosis of malignant primary breast lesions, and these methods cannot replace conventional imaging methods and histologic analysis. However, for the evaluation of primary lesions, PET or PET/CT can be helpful in detecting cancers that are not detected by standard methods because of dense breast lesions or breast implants. This contribution is not the main purpose of using PET or PET/CT essentially. PET provides unique functional information about primary tumors for prognosis and management of disease. FDG-PET has been shown to be of limited value in the staging of axillary lymph node involvement. High PPV of FDG-PET and PET/CT in the diagnosis of axillary lymph node involvement can avoid SNB in some metastatic patients. The current literature shows that FDG-PET and PET/CT have an absolute superiority for the assessment of extra-axillary regional lymph node metastases such as internal mammary, supraclavicular, and mediastinal lymph nodes compared with conventional methods in the initial diagnosis of breast cancer and follow-up. This assessment can change the stage of some patients as well as the therapeutic regimen. At present, FDG-PET is still not an acceptable method for the initial staging of patients with primary breast cancers. However, there is no argument that FDG-PET or PET/CT is the preferred method over conventional imaging studies for assessment of the extent of distant metastatic disease and diagnosis of patients with suspicion of recurrent or metastatic disease. It is well known that the integrated PET/CT systems add morphologic information to functional PET imaging and that this contribution can positively affect the assessment of PET imaging in staging and restaging of patients with breast cancer. Technological developments of PET/CT and PET/MRI systems have a great potential for better diagnosis, staging, and restaging in patients with breast cancer in the near future.

REFERENCES

1. Sant M, Allemani C, Berrino F, et al. European Concerted Action on Survival and Care of Cancer Patients (EUROCARE) Working Group. Breast carcinoma survival in Europe and the United States. Cancer 2004;100(4):715–22.
2. Avril N, Adler LP. F-18 fluorodeoxyglucose-positron emission tomography imaging for primary breast cancer and loco-regional staging. Radiol Clin North Am 2007;45(4):645–57.
3. Kopans DB. The positive predictive value of mammography. AJR Am J Roentgenol 1992; 158(3):521–6.
4. Franceschi D, Crowe J, Zollinger R, et al. Biopsy of the breast for mammographically detected lesions. Surg Gynecol Obstet 1990;171(6):449–55.
5. Skinner MA, Swain M, Simmons R, et al. Nonpalpable breast lesions at biopsy. A detailed analysis of radiographic features. Ann Surg 1988;208(2): 203–8.
6. Kubota K, Matsuzawa T, Amemiya A, et al. Imaging of breast cancer with [18F]fluorodeoxyglucose and positron emission tomography. J Comput Assist Tomogr 1989;13(6):1097–8.
7. Wahl RL, Cody RL, Hutchins GD, et al. Primary and metastatic breast carcinoma: initial clinical evaluation with PET with the radiolabeled glucose analogue 2-[F-18]-fluoro-2-deoxy-D-glucose. Radiology 1991; 179(3):765–70.
8. Adler LP, Crowe JP, al-Kaisi NK, et al. Evaluation of breast masses and axillary lymph nodes with [F-18] 2-deoxy-2-fluoro-D-glucose PET. Radiology 1993;187(3):743–50.
9. Dehdashti F, Mortimer JE, Siegel BA, et al. Positron tomographic assessment of estrogen receptors in breast cancer: comparison with FDG-PET and in vitro receptor assays. J Nucl Med 1995;36(10): 1766–74.
10. Avril N, Rosé CA, Schelling M, et al. Breast imaging with positron emission tomography and fluorine-18 fluorodeoxyglucose: use and limitations. J Clin Oncol 2000;18(20):3495–502.
11. Schirrmeister H, Kühn T, Guhlmann A, et al. Fluorine-18 2-deoxy-2-fluoro-D-glucose PET in the preoperative staging of breast cancer: comparison with the standard staging procedures. Eur J Nucl Med 2001;28(3):351–8.
12. Cermik TF, Mavi A, Basu S, et al. Impact of FDG PET on the preoperative staging of newly diagnosed breast cancer. Eur J Nucl Med Mol Imaging 2008; 35(3):475–83.
13. Amano G, Ohuchi N, Ishibashi T, et al. Correlation of three-dimensional magnetic resonance imaging with precise histopathological map concerning carcinoma extension in the breast. Breast Cancer Res Treat 2000;60(1):43–55.
14. Uematsu T, Kasami M, Yuen S. Comparison of FDG PET and MRI for evaluating the tumor extent of breast cancer and the impact of FDG PET on the systemic staging and prognosis of patients who are candidates for breast-conserving therapy. Breast Cancer 2009;16(2):97–104.
15. Uematsu T, Yuen S, Kasami M, et al. Comparison of magnetic resonance imaging, multidetector row computed tomography, ultrasonography, and mammography for tumor extension of breast cancer. Breast Cancer Res Treat 2008;112(3):461–74.
16. Berg WA, Weinberg IN, Narayanan D, et al. Positron Emission Mammography Working Group. High-resolution fluorodeoxyglucose positron emission tomography with compression ("positron emission mammography") is highly accurate in depicting primary breast cancer. Breast J 2006;12(4):309–23.
17. Eubank WB, Mankoff DA. Evolving role of positron emission tomography in breast cancer imaging. Semin Nucl Med 2005;35(2):84–99.
18. Zhuang H, Pourdehnad M, Lambright ES, et al. Dual time point 18F-FDG PET imaging for differentiating malignant from inflammatory processes. J Nucl Med 2001;42(9):1412–7.
19. Hustinx R, Smith RJ, Benard F, et al. Dual time point fluorine-18 fluorodeoxyglucose positron emission tomography: a potential method to differentiate malignancy from inflammation and normal tissue in the head and neck. Eur J Nucl Med 1999;26(10):1345–8.
20. Beaulieu S, Kinahan P, Tseng J, et al. SUV varies with time after injection in (18)F-FDG PET of breast cancer: characterization and method to adjust for time differences. J Nucl Med 2003;44(7):1044–50.
21. Boerner AR, Weckesser M, Herzog H, et al. Optimal scan time for fluorine-18 fluorodeoxyglucose positron emission tomography in breast cancer. Eur J Nucl Med 1999;26(3):226–30.

22. Mavi A, Urhan M, Yu JQ, et al. Dual time point 18F-FDG PET imaging detects breast cancer with high sensitivity and correlates well with histologic subtypes. J Nucl Med 2006;47(9):1440–6.

23. Yutani K, Tatsumi M, Uehara T, et al. Effect of patients' being prone during FDG PET for the diagnosis of breast cancer. AJR Am J Roentgenol 1999; 173(5):1337–9.

24. Kaida H, Ishibashi M, Fuji T, et al. Improved breast cancer detection of prone breast fluorodeoxyglucose-PET in 118 patients. Nucl Med Commun 2008;29(10):885–93.

25. Siggelkow W, Rath W, Buell U, et al. FDG PET and tumour markers in the diagnosis of recurrent and metastatic breast cancer. Eur J Nucl Med Mol Imaging 2004;31(Suppl 1):S118–24.

26. Fueger BJ, Weber WA, Quon A, et al. Performance of 2-deoxy-2-[F-18]fluoro-D-glucose positron emission tomography and integrated PET/CT in restaged breast cancer patients. Mol Imaging Biol 2005;7(5): 369–76.

27. Imbriaco M, Caprio MG, Limite G, et al. Dual-time-point 18F-FDG PET/CT versus dynamic breast MRI of suspicious breast lesions. AJR Am J Roentgenol 2008;191(5):1323–30.

28. Ranaboldo CJ, Mitchel A, Royle GT, et al. Axillary nodal status in women with screen-detected breast cancer. Eur J Surg Oncol 1993;19(2):130–3.

29. Walls J, Boggis CR, Wilson M, et al. Treatment of the axilla in patients with screen-detected breast cancer. Br J Surg 1993;80(4):436–8.

30. Ververs JM, Roumen RM, Vingerhoets AJ, et al. Risk, severity and predictors of physical and psychological morbidity after axillary lymph node dissection for breast cancer. Eur J Cancer 2001;37(8):991–9.

31. Veronesi U, Paganelli G, Galimberti V, et al. Sentinel-node biopsy to avoid axillary dissection in breast cancer with clinically negative lymph-nodes. Lancet 1997;349(9069):1864–7.

32. Utech CI, Young CS, Winter PF. Prospective evaluation of fluorine-18 fluorodeoxyglucose positron emission tomography in breast cancer for staging of the axilla related to surgery and immunocytochemistry. Eur J Nucl Med 1996;23(12):1588–93.

33. Avril N, Dose J, Jänicke F, et al. Assessment of axillary lymph node involvement in breast cancer patients with positron emission tomography using radiolabeled 2-(fluorine-18)-fluoro-2-deoxy-D-glucose. J Natl Cancer Inst 1996;88(17):1204–9.

34. Adler LP, Faulhaber PF, Schnur KC, et al. Axillary lymph node metastases: screening with [F-18]2-deoxy-2-fluoro-D-glucose (FDG) PET. Radiology 1997;203(2):323–7.

35. Smith IC, Ogston KN, Whitford P, et al. Staging of the axilla in breast cancer: accurate in vivo assessment using positron emission tomography with 2-(fluorine-18)-fluoro-2-deoxy-D-glucose. Ann Surg 1998; 228(2):220–7.

36. Crippa F, Agresti R, Seregni E, et al. Prospective evaluation of fluorine-18-FDG PET in presurgical staging of the axilla in breast cancer. J Nucl Med 1998;39(1):4–8.

37. Rostom AY, Powe J, Kandil A, et al. Positron emission tomography in breast cancer: a clinicopathological correlation of results. Br J Radiol 1999;72(863): 1064–8.

38. Greco M, Crippa F, Agresti R, et al. Axillary lymph node staging in breast cancer by 2-fluoro-2-deoxy-D-glucose-positron emission tomography: clinical evaluation and alternative management. J Natl Cancer Inst 2001;93(8):630–5.

39. van der Hoeven JJ, Hoekstra OS, Comans EF, et al. Determinants of diagnostic performance of [F-18]fluorodeoxyglucose positron emission tomography for axillary staging in breast cancer. Ann Surg 2002;236(5):619–24.

40. Wahl RL, Siegel BA, Coleman RE, et al. Prospective multicenter study of axillary nodal staging by positron emission tomography in breast cancer: a report of the staging breast cancer with PET Study Group. J Clin Oncol 2004;22(2):277–85.

41. Lovrics PJ, Chen V, Coates G, et al. A prospective evaluation of positron emission tomography scanning, sentinel lymph node biopsy, and standard axillary dissection for axillary staging in patients with early stage breast cancer. Ann Surg Oncol 2004; 11(9):846–53.

42. Chung A, Liou D, Karlan S, et al. Preoperative FDG-PET for axillary metastases in patients with breast cancer. Arch Surg 2006;141(8):783–9.

43. Gil-Rendo A, Zornoza G, García-Velloso MJ, et al. Fluorodeoxyglucose positron emission tomography with sentinel lymph node biopsy for evaluation of axillary involvement in breast cancer. Br J Surg 2006;93(6):707–12.

44. Heusner TA, Kuemmel S, Hahn S, et al. Diagnostic value of full-dose FDG PET/CT for axillary lymph node staging in breast cancer patients. Eur J Nucl Med Mol Imaging 2009;36(10):1543–50.

45. Kim J, Lee J, Chang E, et al. Selective sentinel node plus additional non-sentinel node biopsy based on an FDG-PET/CT scan in early breast cancer patients: single institutional experience. World J Surg 2009;33(5):943–9.

46. Veronesi U, Paganelli G, Viale G, et al. A randomized comparison of sentinel-node biopsy with routine axillary dissection in breast cancer. N Engl J Med 2003; 349(6):546–53.

47. Shivers S, Cox C, Leight G, et al. Final results of the department of defense multicenter breast lymphatic mapping trial. Ann Surg Oncol 2002;9(3):248–55.

48. Keskek M, Balas S, Gokoz A, et al. Re-evaluation of axillary skip metastases in the era of sentinel lymph node biopsy in breast cancer. Surg Today 2006; 36(12):1047–52.

49. Donegan WL. The influence of untreated internal mammary metastases upon the course of mammary cancer. Cancer 1977;39(2):533–8.

50. Noguchi M, Ohta N, Thomas M, et al. Risk of internal mammary lymph node metastases and its prognostic value in breast cancer patients. J Surg Oncol 1993;52(1):26–30.

51. Bellon JR, Livingston RB, Eubank WB, et al. Evaluation of the internal mammary lymph nodes by FDG-PET in locally advanced breast cancer (LABC). Am J Clin Oncol 2004;27(4):407–10.

52. Le MG, Arriagada R, de Vathaire F, et al. Can internal mammary chain treatment decrease the risk of death for patients with medial breast cancers and positive axillary lymph nodes? Cancer 1990;66(11):2313–8.

53. Eubank WB, Mankoff DA, Takasugi J, et al. 18Fluorodeoxyglucose positron emission tomography to detect mediastinal or internal mammary metastases in breast cancer. J Clin Oncol 2001;19(15):3516–23.

54. Heusner TA, Kuemmel S, Umutlu L, et al. Breast cancer staging in a single session: whole-body PET/CT mammography. J Nucl Med 2008;49(8):1215–22.

55. Ravaioli A, Pasini G, Polselli A, et al. Staging of breast cancer: new recommended standard procedure. Breast Cancer Res Treat 2002;72(1):53–60.

56. Gerber B, Seitz E, Muller H, et al. Perioperative screening for metastatic disease is not indicated in patients with primary breast cancer and no clinical signs of tumor spread. Breast Cancer Res Treat 2003;82(1):29–37.

57. Schneider C, Fehr MK, Steiner RA, et al. Frequency and distribution pattern of distant metastases in breast cancer patients at the time of primary presentation. Arch Gynecol Obstet 2003;269(1):9–12.

58. Solomayer EF, Diel IJ, Meyberg GC, et al. Metastatic breast cancer: clinical course, prognosis and therapy related to the first site of metastasis. Breast Cancer Res Treat 2000;59(3):271–8.

59. Weir L, Worsley D, Bernstein V. The value of FDG positron emission tomography in the management of patients with breast cancer. Breast J 2005;11(3):204–9.

60. Fuster D, Duch J, Paredes P, et al. Preoperative staging of large primary breast cancer with [18F]fluorodeoxyglucose positron emission tomography/computed tomography compared with conventional imaging procedures. J Clin Oncol 2008;26(29):4746–51.

61. Mahner S, Schirrmacher S, Brenner W, et al. Comparison between positron emission tomography using 2-[fluorine-18]fluoro-2-deoxy-D-glucose, conventional imaging and computed tomography for staging of breast cancer. Ann Oncol 2008;19(7):1249–54.

62. Carkaci S, Macapinlac HA, Cristofanilli M, et al. Retrospective study of 18F-FDG PET/CT in the diagnosis of inflammatory breast cancer: preliminary data. J Nucl Med 2009;50(2):231–8.

63. Cook GJ, Houston S, Rubens R, et al. Detection of bone metastases in breast cancer by 18FDG PET: differing metabolic activity in osteoblastic and osteolytic lesions. J Clin Oncol 1998;16(10):3375–9.

64. Martin TJ, Moseley JM. Mechanisms in the skeletal complications of breast cancer. Endocr Relat Cancer 2000;7(4):271–84.

65. Maffioli L, Florimonte L, Pagani L, et al. Current role of bone scan with phosphonates in the follow-up of breast cancer. Eur J Nucl Med Mol Imaging 2004;31(Suppl 1):S143–8.

66. Rosenthal DI. Radiologic diagnosis of bone metastases. Cancer 1997;80(Suppl 8):1595–607.

67. Ohta M, Tokuda Y, Suzuki Y, et al. Whole body PET for the evaluation of bony metastases in patients with breast cancer: comparison with 99Tcm-MDP bone scintigraphy. Nucl Med Commun 2001;22(8):875–9.

68. Yang SN, Liang JA, Lin FJ, et al. Comparing whole body (18)F-2-deoxyglucose positron emission tomography and technetium-99m methylene diphosphonate bone scan to detect bone metastases in patients with breast cancer. J Cancer Res Clin Oncol 2002;128(6):325–8.

69. Moon DH, Maddahi J, Silverman DH, et al. Accuracy of whole-body fluorine-18-FDG PET for the detection of recurrent or metastatic breast carcinoma. J Nucl Med 1998;39(3):431–5.

70. Kao CH, Hsieh JF, Tsai SC, et al. Comparison and discrepancy of 18F-2-deoxyglucose positron emission tomography and Tc-99m MDP bone scan to detect bone metastases. Anticancer Res 2000;20(3B):2189–92.

71. Abe K, Sasaki M, Kuwabara Y, et al. Comparison of 18FDG-PET with 99mTc-HMDP scintigraphy for the detection of bone metastases in patients with breast cancer. Ann Nucl Med 2005;19(7):573–9.

72. Nakai T, Okuyama C, Kubota T, et al. Pitfalls of FDG-PET for the diagnosis of osteoblastic bone metastases in patients with breast cancer. Eur J Nucl Med Mol Imaging 2005;32(11):1253–8.

73. Yamashita K, Koyama H, Inaji H. Prognostic significance of bone metastasis from breast cancer. Clin Orthop Relat Res 1995;312:89–94.

74. Clarke M, Collins R, Darby S, et al. Early Breast Cancer Trialists' Collaborative Group (EBCTCG). Effects of radiotherapy and of differences in the extent of surgery for early breast cancer on local recurrence and 15-year survival: an overview of the randomized trials. Lancet 2005;366(9503):2087–106.

75. Khatcheressian JL, Wolff AC, Smith TJ, et al. American Society of Clinical Oncology. American Society of Clinical Oncology 2006 update of the breast

cancer follow-up and management guidelines in the adjuvant setting. J Clin Oncol 2006;24(31):5091–7.

76. Mankoff DA, Eubank WB. Current and future use of positron emission tomography (PET) in breast cancer. J Mammary Gland Biol Neoplasia 2006; 11(2):125–36.

77. Gallowitsch HJ, Kresnik E, Gasser J, et al. F-18 fluorodeoxyglucose positron-emission tomography in the diagnosis of tumor recurrence and metastases in the follow-up of patients with breast carcinoma: a comparison to conventional imaging. Invest Radiol 2003;38(5):250–6.

78. Wolfort RM, Li BD, Johnson LW, et al. The role of whole-body fluorine-18-FDG positron emission tomography in the detection of recurrence in symptomatic patients with stages II and III breast cancer. World J Surg 2006;30(8):1422–7.

79. Molina R, Zanón G, Filella X, et al. Use of serial carcinoembryonic antigen and CA 15.3 assays in detecting relapses in breast cancer patients. Breast Cancer Res Treat 1995;36(1):41–8.

80. Liu CS, Shen YY, Lin CC, et al. Clinical impact of [(18)F]FDG-PET in patients with suspected recurrent breast cancer based on asymptomatically elevated tumor marker serum levels: a preliminary report. Jpn J Clin Oncol 2002;32(7):244–7.

81. Suárez M, Pérez-Castejón MJ, Jiménez A, et al. Early diagnosis of recurrent breast cancer with FDG-PET in patients with progressive elevation of serum tumor markers. Q J Nucl Med 2002;46(2):113–21.

82. Kluetz PG, Meltzer CC, Villemagne VL, et al. Combined PET/CT imaging in oncology. Impact on patient management. Clin Positron Imaging 2000; 3(6):223–30.

83. Eubank WB, Mankoff DA, Schmiedl UP, et al. Imaging of oncologic patients: benefit of combined CT and FDG PET in the diagnosis of malignancy. AJR Am J Roentgenol 1998;171(4):1103–10.

84. Bar-Shalom R, Yefremov N, Guralnik L, et al. Clinical performance of PET/CT in evaluation of cancer: additional value for diagnostic imaging and patient management. J Nucl Med 2003;44(8):1200–9.

85. Piperkova E, Raphael B, Altinyay ME, et al. Impact of PET/CT in comparison with same day contrast enhanced CT in breast cancer management. Clin Nucl Med 2007;32(6):429–34.

86. Tatsumi M, Cohade C, Mourtzikos KA, et al. Initial experience with FDG-PET/CT in the evaluation of breast cancer. Eur J Nucl Med Mol Imaging 2006;33(3):254–62.

87. Radan L, Ben-Haim S, Bar-Shalom R, et al. The role of FDG-PET/CT in suspected recurrence of breast cancer. Cancer 2006;107(11):2545–51.

Index

Note: Page numbers of article titles are in **boldface** type.

A

[^{11}C]-Acetate, for breast cancer, 375
[^{18}F]-AH111585, for breast cancer, 372
American College of Radiology Imaging Network, contralateral breast imaging trials of, 344
Amino acids, labeled, for breast cancer treatment monitoring, 365, 375
Angiogenesis, tumor, PET imaging of, 371–372
[^{99m}Tc]-Annexin, for breast cancer, 376
Apoptosis, in breast cancer, 375–376

B

Bevacizumab, 371
Bombesin, labeled, for breast cancer, 334–335
Breast cancer
  chemotherapy for
    novel tracers, 371–376
    response monitoring in, **359–369**
  contralateral breast screening in, **343–347**
  diagnosis of, 391–394
  follow-up imaging in, **391–404**
  lymph node status in, 394–396
  magnetic resonance spectroscopy for, 375
  mammography for, **317–327**
  metastasis of. *See* Metastasis.
  MRI for, 343–344, 359
  multimodality imaging in, 324–325
  PET/CT for. *See* PET/CT.
  PET for. *See* PET.
  radiation planning for, **349–357**
  receptor imaging in, **329–341**, 373–375
  recurrent, 353, 397–400
  staging of, 394–396
  surgery for, radiation planning after, 351–353
  tumor biology studies in, **381–389**
Breast conserving surgery, radiation planning after, PET/CT for, 351
British-Columbia Cancer Agency, postmastectomy studies of, 351–352

C

Cell lines, breast cancer, PET studies of, 388
Chemotherapy, for breast cancer, response monitoring in
  novel tracers for, 371–376
  PET/CT for, **359–369**
Choline, labeled, for breast cancer, 375
Clear-PEM instrument, 322

Contralateral breast screening, **343–347**
  MRI for, 343–344
  PET and PET/CT for, 344–346
Crystal Clear Collaboration, PEM instrument of, 322
CT, PET with. *See* PET/CT.

D

Deformable registration, in multimodality imaging, 324
[^{99m}Tc]-Depreotide, for breast cancer, 334

E

Estradiol, labeled, for breast cancer, 330, 373–374
Estrogen antagonist imaging, for breast cancer, 333
Estrogen receptor imaging, for breast cancer, 330–332, 373–375, 382, 384
European Organisation for Research and Treatment of Cancer, postmastectomy studies of, 351

F

FDG. *See* [^{18}F]-2-Fluoro-2-deoxy-D-glucose.
Flare phenomenon, in PET, after treatment, 364–365
[^{18}F]-2-Fluoro-2-deoxy-D-glucose, for breast cancer, 331–332
  contralateral breast, 344–346
  correlation with other parameters, 387–388
  disease burden and, 384–385
  for cell line studies, 388
  for diagnosis, 391–394
  for radiation planning, 349–357
  for staging, **391–404**
  history of, 383
  hormone receptor expression and, 382, 384
  mammography, 318
  recurrent, 397–400
  treatment monitoring, 360–365
  tumor biology and, **381–389**
  tumor perfusion, 372, 375
  tumor proliferation index and, 385–387
  tumor subtype and, 381–382
[^{18}F]-2-Fluoroestradiol, for breast cancer, 330–332, 373–374
16ß-Fluoromoxestrol, for breast cancer, 330–331
[^{18}F]-Fluoropaclitaxel, for breast cancer, 373
[^{18}F]-Fluorotamoxifen, for breast cancer, 333
[^{18}F]-Fluorothymidine, for breast cancer, 365, 375
Fulvestrant, labeled, for breast cancer, 333

doi:10.1016/S1556-8598(09)00182-5
1556-8598/09/$ – see front matter © 2009 Elsevier Inc. All rights reserved.

Moving?

Make sure your subscription moves with you!

To notify us of your new address, find your **Clinics Account Number** (located on your mailing label above your name), and contact customer service at:

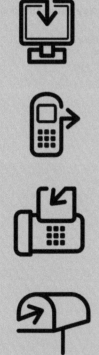

Email: journalscustomerservice-usa@elsevier.com

800-654-2452 (subscribers in the U.S. & Canada)
314-447-8871 (subscribers outside of the U.S. & Canada)

Fax number: 314-447-8029

Elsevier Health Sciences Division
Subscription Customer Service
3251 Riverport Lane
Maryland Heights, MO 63043

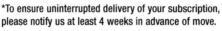

*To ensure uninterrupted delivery of your subscription, please notify us at least 4 weeks in advance of move.

ELSEVIER

Printed and bound by CPI Group (UK) Ltd, Croydon, CR0 4YY

03/10/2024

01040352-0011